SpringerBriefs in Modern Perspectives on Disability Research

This book series on disability research is a comprehensive collection of research on disability and related issues. The series is designed to promote interdisciplinary collaboration and exchange, bringing together scholars and practitioners from different fields to share their perspectives and insights. Disability research is an interdisciplinary field that examines the social, cultural, historical, and political dimensions of disability. It encompasses a wide range of topics, including disability rights, accessibility, assistive technologies, healthcare, education, employment, and social welfare. Disability research scholars employ a range of theoretical and methodological approaches to understand the experiences of people with disabilities, as well as the ways in which disability intersects with other social identities such as race, gender, sexuality, and class.

The series seeks to advance knowledge and understanding of disability by publishing rigorous, innovative, and relevant research. It aims to promote disability rights and social justice by highlighting the ways in which people with disabilities are marginalized and discriminated against in society, and advocating for greater social inclusion and accessibility. The series also seeks to inform policy and practice by disseminating research findings that can help to shape policy decisions and contribute to positive social change.

Khoiruddin Bashori • Zalik Nuryana

Disability Inclusion

Integrating Islamic Perspectives in Education

Springer

Khoiruddin Bashori
Department of Psychology
Universitas Ahmad Dahlan
Yogyakarta, Indonesia

Zalik Nuryana
Department of Islamic Education
Universitas Ahmad Dahlan
Yogyakarta, Indonesia

ISSN 3004-9709 ISSN 3004-9717 (electronic)
SpringerBriefs in Modern Perspectives on Disability Research
ISBN 978-981-95-8906-7 ISBN 978-981-95-8907-4 (eBook)
https://doi.org/10.1007/978-981-95-8907-4

This Springer imprint is published by the registered company Springer Nature Singapore Pte Ltd.
The registered company address is: 152 Beach Road, #21-01/04 Gateway East, Singapore 189721, Singapore

Preface

In recent decades, disability inclusion has become a defining concern in global educational reform, human rights discourse, and social justice movements. Within Muslim societies, however, inclusive education continues to encounter conceptual, cultural, and institutional challenges that require contextually grounded ethical responses. This book, Disability Inclusion: Integrating Islamic Perspectives in Education, seeks to address this gap by offering a comprehensive exploration of disability inclusion through the lens of Islamic moral theology, educational philosophy, and contemporary inclusive practice. Rather than approaching inclusion solely as a policy or technical endeavor, this volume frames it as a moral and spiritual responsibility rooted in Islamic values of dignity, justice, compassion, and collective obligation. By doing so, the book contributes to an emerging body of scholarship that bridges Islamic intellectual traditions with modern educational and disability studies.

The motivation for this book arises from the persistent tension between Islamic ethical ideals and lived social realities in many Muslim-majority contexts. While Islamic teachings uphold the inherent dignity of all human beings, persons with disabilities often continue to experience stigma, marginalization, and limited access to educational opportunities. This contradiction calls for deeper scholarly engagement that moves beyond legalistic or charitable responses toward structural and pedagogical transformation. The chapters assembled in this volume aim to critically examine how Islamic theology, jurisprudence, and moral philosophy can provide robust normative foundations for inclusive education. At the same time, the book engages contemporary research in inclusive pedagogy, disability studies, and educational technology to offer practical pathways for implementation within schools, religious institutions, and communities.

This book is structured to guide readers from foundational ethical principles toward concrete educational praxis. Chapter 1 establishes the theological and moral underpinnings of inclusion by examining Qurʾānic ethics, Prophetic traditions, and the objectives of Islamic law (*maqāṣid al-sharīʿah*). It articulates how concepts such as *karāmah* (human dignity), *ʿadl* (justice), *raḥmah* (compassion), and *masʾūliyyah* (moral accountability) form an ontological and ethical basis for recognizing the full moral status of persons with disabilities. This foundational chapter provides the conceptual vocabulary and theological legitimacy upon which subsequent discussions of pedagogy, technology, and community transformation are built.

Chapter 2 turns to the social and cultural dimensions of disability in Muslim communities. It critically explores how inherited beliefs, local traditions, and informal religious narratives sometimes perpetuate stigma, despite clear theological prohibitions against discrimination and mockery. By analyzing the gap between normative Islamic ethics and everyday social practices, the chapter highlights the urgent need for cultural critique and ethical reorientation. This discussion sets the stage for understanding inclusion not merely as individual goodwill, but as the dismantling of structural and attitudinal barriers embedded in family life, community expectations, and institutional routines.

The pedagogical heart of the book appears in Chap. 3, which focuses on curriculum adaptation and instructional strategies in Islamic Religious Education. Drawing on case studies and classroom-based evidence, this chapter demonstrates how multisensory methods, differentiated content, and individualized learning plans enable students with disabilities to engage meaningfully with religious knowledge and practice. The chapter emphasizes that inclusive pedagogy is not an educational concession, but an enactment of Islamic justice in learning. It offers practical models for teachers, school leaders, and curriculum designers seeking to align religious instruction with ethical commitments to equity and participation.

Chapter 4 extends the discussion into the digital domain by examining assistive technologies, Universal Design for Learning (UDL), and digital accessibility in Islamic education. As digital platforms increasingly mediate religious learning, ensuring equitable technological access becomes a moral imperative. This chapter explores how screen readers, audio Qur'ān applications, speech-to-text tools, and accessible learning management systems enhance intellectual and spiritual agency for learners with disabilities. It situates technological inclusion within the maqāṣid framework, showing that protecting intellect, dignity, and well-being in digital spaces is an extension of Islamic ethical responsibility.

Recognizing that sustainable inclusion cannot be achieved through schools alone, Chap. 5 highlights the transformative role of families, mosques, and Islamic educational institutions as interconnected community environments. It illustrates how parental advocacy, mosque accessibility initiatives, leadership commitment, and inclusive pesantren models in Indonesia contribute to shifting communal attitudes and practices. By presenting community-based inclusion as collective moral work, this chapter demonstrates that embedding Islamic ethical values in everyday social spaces is essential for reducing stigma and enabling genuine participation for persons with disabilities.

Chapter 6 completes the thematic arc of the book by examining spiritual formation and moral development in inclusive Islamic education. It presents qualitative evidence showing that adapted religious instruction not only supports academic learning but also nurtures empathy, resilience, ethical awareness, and spiritual confidence among students with disabilities. Prophetic traditions that frame disability as a test of faith and a means of spiritual elevation are reinterpreted as sources of hope, patience, and gratitude rather than justification for passivity or exclusion. This chapter ultimately positions inclusive religious education as a pathway to moral flourishing for all learners.

Throughout the volume, the contributors adopt an interdisciplinary approach that integrates Islamic studies, education, disability research, sociology, and digital pedagogy. This synthesis reflects the book's central conviction: that inclusive education in Muslim contexts must be simultaneously theologically grounded, pedagogically sound, and socially transformative. Rather than importing external models uncritically, the book seeks to generate indigenous frameworks of inclusion that resonate with Islamic intellectual heritage while remaining responsive to contemporary educational realities and international inclusion standards.

This book is intended for scholars, educators, religious leaders, policymakers, disability advocates, and students interested in Islamic education and inclusive practice. It invites readers to rethink disability inclusion not as a marginal topic but as a core expression of Islamic moral vision and social responsibility. By aligning theological ethics, community engagement, and institutional reform, the volume offers a sustainable roadmap toward educational environments where dignity is honored, justice is enacted, compassion is lived, and participation is universal. It is our hope that this work will inspire continued research, dialogue, and action toward building inclusive societies in which every learner can belong, contribute, and flourish.

25 March 2026

Yogyakarta, Indonesia — Khoiruddin Bashori
Yogyakarta, Indonesia — Zalik Nuryana

Contents

Chapter 1
Foundations of Islamic Inclusion: Values and Principles

Abstract This chapter develops an Islamic ethical framework for inclusive education by grounding inclusion within Qurʾānic moral theology and the objectives of Islamic law (*maqāṣid al-sharīʿah*). While inclusive education is commonly framed through secular human rights and policy discourses, the chapter argues that Islamic moral traditions offer a coherent and internally grounded foundation for educational inclusion, particularly for learners with disabilities. Drawing on key Qurʾānic principles: human dignity (*karāmah al-insān*), justice (*ʿadl*), mercy (*raḥmah*), diversity (*taʿāruf*), and moral accountability (*masʾūliyyah*) the chapter demonstrates that disability is understood not as deficiency or punishment but as part of divinely intended human diversity. The discussion situates inclusion within the maqāṣid framework, emphasizing the protection of intellect, life, and honor as ethical imperatives requiring equitable educational access. By linking moral theology with educational praxis, inclusion is conceptualized as a form of collective moral responsibility (*ʿibādah ijtimāʿiyyah*) rather than a peripheral policy adaptation.

Keywords Inclusive Islamic Education · Disability & Human Dignity · Qurʾānic Ethics · *Maqāṣid al-Sharīʿah* · Educational Justice

1.1 Introduction

Inclusive education has become a central theme in contemporary educational research and policy, particularly in relation to equity, human rights, and sustainable development. International frameworks such as the United Nations Convention on the Rights of Persons with Disabilities and the UNESCO Global Education Monitoring Report position inclusion as a structural and ethical requirement of modern education systems (United Nations, 2016; UNESCO, 2020). Despite this growing consensus, dominant models of inclusive education are largely articulated within secular human rights and policy-oriented paradigms. In Muslim-majority contexts, this has resulted in a conceptual gap between global inclusion discourse

K. Bashori, Z. Nuryana, *Disability Inclusion*, SpringerBriefs in Modern Perspectives on Disability Research,
https://doi.org/10.1007/978-981-95-8907-4_1

and locally meaningful ethical frameworks. As a consequence, inclusive education is sometimes perceived as externally driven rather than normatively grounded within Islamic intellectual and moral traditions.

Islamic moral theology offers a comprehensive ethical worldview that can meaningfully contribute to contemporary debates on inclusion. Foundational concepts such as human dignity (*karāmah al-insān*), justice (*ʿadl*), mercy (*raḥmah*), and moral accountability (*masʾūliyyah*) are deeply embedded in the Qurʾān and Prophetic tradition and have been extensively developed in classical and contemporary Islamic scholarship (Kamali, 2021a, 2021b; Abou El Fadl, 2022). These principles articulate a vision of humanity that affirms inherent worth, moral agency, and social responsibility irrespective of physical ability or social status. However, the application of these ethical foundations to educational inclusion, particularly in relation to disability, remains under-theorized within Islamic educational studies, creating a disjunction between normative theology and lived educational practice.

Disability presents a critical lens through which this ethical gap becomes visible. While Islamic sources reject associations between disability and moral deficiency, cultural practices in some Muslim societies continue to reflect stigma, exclusion, and deficit-based assumptions (Bazna & Hatab, 2022; Ghaly, 2022). Contemporary scholarship in inclusive education emphasizes that exclusion is primarily produced by social, institutional, and attitudinal barriers rather than individual imIErment (Florian, 2019; Slee, 2023). When read through an Islamic ethical framework, Qurʾānic narratives and legal-ethical principles offer strong normative support for equity, accommodation, and participatory belonging. This convergence suggests significant potential for dialogue between Islamic moral theology and contemporary inclusion theory.

This chapter seeks to articulate an Islamic ethical foundation for inclusive education by systematically examining Qurʾānic principles, Islamic moral theology, and the objectives of Islamic law (*maqāṣid al-sharīʿah*). Rather than proposing inclusion as a policy adaptation or charitable response, the chapter conceptualizes it as a moral and ethical imperative intrinsic to the Islamic worldview. The discussion progresses from foundational ethical concepts: dignity, justice, mercy, diversity, and accountability to their implications for educational praxis. By doing so, the chapter contributes to Islamic educational scholarship and inclusive education studies, positioning inclusion as an authentic and normatively grounded expression of Islamic moral vision.

1.2 Human Dignity (*Karāmah al-Insān*) as the Ontological Basis of Inclusion

Islamic inclusion is fundamentally grounded in the Qurʾānic concept of *karāmah al-insān* (human dignity), which affirms the inherent worth of every human being by virtue of divine creation. The verse "And indeed We have honored the children of

Adam" (Qurʾān 17:70) establishes dignity as an ontological given, independent of physical ability, cognitive capacity, productivity, or social recognition. Contemporary Islamic scholarship emphasizes that this dignity is universal and unconditional, encompassing all forms of human diversity, including disability (Kamali, 2021a, 2021b). From this perspective, disability does not diminish human value but reflects the plurality of God's creation. Such an understanding challenges utilitarian and ableist frameworks that implicitly rank human worth based on functional performance.

Classical and modern Islamic thinkers consistently assert that dignity precedes all social categorization and evaluative labeling. Human beings are honored not for what they can produce, but for who they are as moral and spiritual agents (*mukallaf*) endowed with responsibility and consciousness (Ghaly, 2019). This ontological equality directly contests deficit-based conceptions of disability that dominate many contemporary educational systems. Islamic anthropology views imIErment as morally neutral and unrelated to divine favor or disfavor. Therefore, exclusionary educational practices contradict the Islamic worldview by implicitly conditioning dignity on normative standards of ability, thereby undermining the Qurʾānic affirmation of equal human worth (Bazna & Hatab, 2020).

In educational contexts, *karāmah al-insān* requires a fundamental ethical reorientation toward learners with disabilities. Students with disabilities must be recognized not as passive recipients of charity or special treatment, but as full subjects of rights, responsibilities, and agency within the learning community (UNESCO, 2020). Islamic ethics frames inclusion as a matter of justice (*ʿadl*) and trust (*amānah*), obligating institutions to remove structural barriers that limit participation. When access to education is denied or restricted, it constitutes not only a policy failure but also a moral violation of God-given dignity. Thus, inclusive education becomes an ethical imperative rooted in Islamic moral theology rather than optional benevolence.

Grounding inclusion in *karāmah al-insān* provides Muslim societies with a robust theological and moral framework for inclusive education. Rather than relying solely on international conventions or legal compliance, Islamic inclusion is framed as alignment with divine intent and moral responsibility (Kamali, 2021a, 2021b). This perspective strengthens the legitimacy of inclusive practices within religious communities and educational institutions. By integrating theology, ethics, and pedagogy, Islamic education can promote models of inclusion that honor diversity while fostering social cohesion. Ultimately, affirming human dignity as ontological reinforces the principle that educational inclusion is not merely a social policy, but a religious and moral obligation grounded in Islam's vision of humanity.

1.3 Justice (ʿAdl) and Equity as Ethical Imperatives

Justice (*ʿadl*) occupies a central position in Islamic moral philosophy and is repeatedly emphasized in the Qurʾān as a binding ethical obligation. The command to "stand firmly for justice" even against personal or social interests (Qurʾān 4:135) frames justice as an active moral responsibility rather than a passive legal ideal. Contemporary Islamic ethics interpret *ʿadl* as requiring contextual and relational fairness, acknowledging unequal starting points among individuals (Kamali, 2021a, 2021b). When applied to inclusion, justice extends beyond formal equality toward substantive equity, ensuring that social arrangements do not perpetuate disadvantage. Within this framework, disability is understood not as personal deficiency but as a condition that necessitates ethical responsiveness from institutions and communities.

In educational settings, Islamic justice does not imply identical treatment of all learners, but rather fair treatment that enables each student to access learning meaningfully. Islamic jurisprudence articulates this distinction through the principle that equality does not mean sameness (*al-musāwāh lā taʿnī al-tamāthul*), recognizing diversity in human capacities and circumstances (Hallaq, 2019). Consequently, differentiated instruction, reasonable accommodation, and individualized support are not exceptions to justice but expressions of it. Providing assistive technologies, curriculum modifications, or alternative assessment methods for students with disabilities aligns with the ethical demand to remove barriers that obstruct learning and personal development (UNESCO, 2020).

Framing inclusion through *ʿadl* challenges narratives that portray inclusive education as burdensome, costly, or preferential. Islamic ethics rejects the notion that equity-oriented practices constitute unfair advantage, emphasizing instead that justice requires compensating for structural inequality (Kamali, 2021a, 2021b). When educational systems ignore differences in ability or access, they implicitly privilege dominant norms and reproduce exclusion. In this sense, failure to accommodate learners with disabilities represents a form of injustice (*ẓulm*), as it denies individuals their rightful opportunities. Inclusive practices, therefore, function as ethical corrections that restore balance and fairness within educational institutions rather than as discretionary acts of goodwill.

Ultimately, justice-based inclusion situates disability rights within a moral and spiritual framework that resonates deeply in Muslim societies. Rather than relying solely on external legal mandates, Islamic justice provides an internal ethical rationale for transforming educational systems (Ghaly, 2022). By grounding equity in *ʿadl*, inclusion becomes a religious obligation tied to accountability before God. This perspective strengthens institutional commitment to inclusive education by framing it as a fulfillment of moral duty. Justice-oriented inclusion thus aligns Islamic values with contemporary educational ethics, promoting systems that are not only accessible but also morally coherent and socially responsible.

1.4 Mercy (*Raḥmah*) as a Pedagogical Ethos

Mercy (*raḥmah*) is a defining attribute of God in Islam and a foundational principle of Prophetic pedagogy. The Qurʾān describes the Prophet Muḥammad ﷺ as "a mercy to all worlds" (Qurʾān 21:107), highlighting compassion as central to his moral and educational mission. Contemporary Islamic scholars emphasize that raḥmah is not merely an emotional disposition but an ethical orientation that guides social and pedagogical relationships (Kamali, 2022a, 2022b). In the Prophet's educational practice, mercy was expressed through patience, attentiveness to individual differences, and responsiveness to learners' capacities. This Prophetic model offers a normative framework for inclusive education, positioning compassion as an essential pedagogical virtue rather than an optional interpersonal quality.

In pedagogical terms, *raḥmah* extends beyond kindness or sympathy and manifests as a deliberate commitment to learners' holistic well-being. Islamic educational ethics require educators to attend to the emotional, psychological, and social dimensions of learning, particularly for students with disabilities who are vulnerable to exclusion and internalized stigma (Ghaly, 2022). A merciful pedagogy recognizes that learning is inseparable from emotional safety and relational trust. Educators guided by *raḥmah* actively seek to reduce anxiety, shame, and fear within learning environments, fostering a sense of belonging and respect. Such environments allow students with disabilities to engage authentically without feeling merely tolerated or conditionally accepted.

The pedagogical ethos of *raḥmah* resonates strongly with contemporary psychological and educational theories that emphasize trauma-informed, learner-centered, and inclusive approaches. Research in educational psychology underscores that compassion, relational attunement, and emotional support significantly enhance motivation, engagement, and cognitive development, especially among marginalized learners (UNESCO, 2020). Islamic pedagogy anticipates these insights by framing education as a relational and ethical process rather than a purely technical transmission of knowledge. By prioritizing care and understanding, *raḥmah*-based pedagogy challenges rigid, performance-driven educational cultures that often marginalize students who do not conform to normative standards of ability or achievement.

For learners with disabilities, educational environments grounded in *raḥmah* are essential for both academic participation and holistic development. Mercy-oriented inclusion shifts the focus from remediation of deficits to affirmation of personhood and potential (Kamali, 2022a, 2022b). Such environments empower learners to develop confidence, resilience, and agency while fostering mutual empathy among peers. In Islamic educational thought, mercy functions as a moral compass that ensures justice and dignity are enacted in daily pedagogical practice. Ultimately, inclusion rooted in *raḥmah* reflects Islam's vision of education as a humane, relational, and transformative endeavor aligned with spiritual and ethical growth.

1.5 Qurʾānic Ethics of Diversity and Mutual Recognition

Sūra al-Ḥujurāt presents a comprehensive ethical framework for social relations grounded in unity, dignity, and moral accountability. Verses 10–13 affirm that human diversity is divinely intended and purposeful, expressed through the concept of *li-taʿārafū* (that you may come to know one another). Contemporary *Qurʾānic* scholarship emphasizes that this principle establishes diversity as a moral resource rather than a social problem (Abou El Fadl, 2022). Although the verses explicitly reference ethnic and tribal distinctions, their ethical logic extends to all forms of human difference, including disability. From this perspective, variation in human ability is part of God's creative wisdom, calling for ethical engagement rather than hierarchy or exclusion.

The Qurʾānic prohibition against mockery, ridicule, defamation, and negative labeling (Qurʾān 49:11) carries profound implications for inclusive education. These injunctions address not only overt acts of discrimination but also subtle forms of symbolic violence that marginalize vulnerable individuals (Saeed, 2020). In educational environments, stigmatizing language, lowered expectations, or social isolation of learners with disabilities directly contradict these ethical commands. Islamic ethics thus demands vigilance against everyday practices that reproduce exclusion under the guise of normalcy. Inclusion, from this Qurʾānic perspective, is not limited to physical access or policy compliance but requires moral discipline in speech, attitudes, and interpersonal relations.

Qurʾānic ethics also emphasize mutual recognition (*taʿāruf*) as an active, relational process rather than passive tolerance. Mutual recognition requires acknowledging difference without reducing individuals to their differences (Kamali, 2021a, 2021b). Within educational contexts, this principle calls for learning cultures that affirm diversity while resisting deficit-based narratives. Learners with disabilities should be recognized as contributors to collective learning, not merely accommodated participants. Such recognition fosters reciprocal respect and shared responsibility among students and educators. By embedding mutual recognition into pedagogical practice, schools can cultivate environments where diversity is normalized and valued as part of the communal learning experience.

Ultimately, the ethical vision articulated in *Sūra al-Ḥujurāt* positions inclusion as an expression of Qurʾānic social harmony (*iṣlāḥ ijtimāʿī*). Education becomes a key site for actualizing this harmony by shaping attitudes, norms, and relationships (Abou El Fadl, 2022). Inclusive education grounded in Qurʾānic ethics seeks not only to integrate learners with disabilities but to transform social relations within educational institutions. By fostering respect, restraint, and recognition, these principles offer a moral blueprint for inclusive communities. In this framework, inclusion is both a spiritual obligation and a social practice aligned with Islam's broader vision of ethical coexistence.

1.6 Moral Accountability and Disability Awareness

The revelation of *Sūra ʿAbasa:* 1–10 offers a profound ethical lesson on attentiveness, humility, and moral accountability in relation to disability. The Qurʾān's gentle reproach of the Prophet Muḥammad ﷺ for momentarily overlooking Ibn Umm

Maktūm, a blind companion seeking guidance, underscores the seriousness with which Islam treats inclusion and ethical awareness. Contemporary Qurʾānic scholarship emphasizes that this reproach does not diminish the Prophet's status but elevates the moral standard for all believers (Saeed, 2020). Physical imlErment is clearly decoupled from spiritual or intellectual worth, reinforcing the principle that access to knowledge and recognition must never be conditioned on sensory ability, social influence, or outward appearance.

Exegetical analyses of *Sūra ʿAbasa* highlight its role in reorienting social hierarchies and moral priorities. Classical and modern commentators note that the passage shifts attention away from elite listeners toward those who demonstrate sincerity, openness, and moral receptivity (Abou El Fadl, 2022). The blind companion is presented as fully capable of engaging with revelation, thereby dismantling assumptions that equate disability with deficiency. This ethical reversal has enduring relevance for educational contexts, where learners are often implicitly ranked based on perceived ability, confidence, or social capital. Qurʾānic ethics thus challenge educational practices that prioritize visibility, performance, or status over genuine engagement and moral worth.

The moral implications of this narrative extend beyond interpersonal conduct to institutional responsibility. Neglecting learners with disabilities whether through inattention, lowered expectations, or systemic exclusion constitutes a form of ethical failure (*taqṣīr*) in Islamic moral reasoning (Kamali, 2021a, 2021b). Educational leaders and teachers are entrusted with *masʾūliyyah* (moral responsibility) to ensure that no learner is rendered invisible within learning environments. This responsibility includes proactive efforts to recognize diverse learning needs, create accessible pedagogies, and cultivate inclusive cultures. Failure to do so represents not merely administrative oversight but a breach of ethical accountability before God.

As a foundational Qurʾānic narrative, *Sūra ʿAbasa* provides a normative framework for disability awareness in Islamic education. It establishes attentiveness (*iltifāt*), humility, and ethical responsiveness as core virtues of teaching and leadership. By foregrounding the dignity and agency of a person with disability, the text offers a moral blueprint for inclusive educational practice grounded in revelation rather than policy alone (Ghaly, 2022). Inclusion, therefore, emerges as an expression of moral consciousness and accountability. This Qurʾānic ethic invites educators to continually examine whose voices are heard, whose needs are prioritized, and whose presence is overlooked within educational systems.

1.7 Inclusion within the Framework of *Maqāṣid al-Sharīʿah*

The objectives of Islamic law (*maqāṣid al-Sharīʿah*) provide a comprehensive ethical–legal framework for understanding inclusion as a normative obligation rather than a discretionary policy choice. Contemporary maqāṣid scholarship emphasizes that Islamic law is fundamentally concerned with securing human welfare and preventing harm in changing social contexts (Auda, 2021). Within this framework, inclusion aligns with the higher purposes of the *Sharīʿah* by ensuring that social institutions serve the dignity and flourishing of all members of society. Educational exclusion of learners with disabilities contradicts this ethical vision, as it obstructs access to essential capabilities. Thus, inclusion emerges as an expression of legal intentionality (*maqṣūd al-shāriʿ*) grounded in justice, compassion, and public benefit.

Protecting the intellect (*ḥifẓ al-ʿaql*) occupies a central place within the maqāṣid framework and directly implicates educational access and quality. Islamic legal theory recognizes knowledge acquisition as both a right and a communal obligation (*farḍ kifāyah*), making equitable education a moral necessity (Kamali, 2021a, 2021b). When learners with disabilities are denied appropriate educational opportunities, their intellectual development is constrained, undermining this core objective. Inclusive education, through differentiated instruction and accessible learning environments, fulfills *ḥifẓ al-ʿaql* by enabling all learners to cultivate reasoning, understanding, and critical reflection. From a *maqāṣid* perspective, such accommodations are not concessions but essential mechanisms for realizing intellectual justice.

The objectives of protecting life (*ḥifẓ al-nafs*) and honor (*ḥifẓ al-ʿirḍ*) further reinforce the ethical imperative of inclusion. Contemporary Islamic ethics interprets *ḥifẓ al-nafs* to include psychological well-being, emotional security, and freedom from harm, not merely physical survival (Ghaly, 2022). Educational exclusion often produces stress, marginalization, and long-term psychosocial harm for learners with disabilities. Likewise, *ḥifẓ al-ʿirḍ* obligates institutions to prevent stigmatization, labeling, and discriminatory practices that erode personal dignity. Inclusive educational environments therefore function as protective spaces that uphold both emotional integrity and social honor, aligning institutional practice with Islamic moral objectives.

Viewed through the lens of *maqāṣid al-Sharīʿah*, inclusion is not a peripheral concern but a central requirement of Islamic governance and institutional ethics. Educational inclusion serves the public interest (*maṣlaḥah ʿāmmah*) by promoting social cohesion, reducing inequality, and enabling full civic participation (Auda, 2021). Framing inclusion as *maṣlaḥah* strengthens its legitimacy within Islamic jurisprudence and policy discourse, particularly in Muslim-majority contexts. This approach bridges normative Islamic legal theory with contemporary human rights and inclusive education frameworks. Ultimately, *maqāṣid*-based inclusion affirms that equitable education is both a moral duty and a legal responsibility rooted in the higher purposes of the *Sharīʿah*.

1.8 From Moral Theology to Educational Praxis

The final thematic movement of this chapter bridges Islamic moral theology with concrete educational praxis, emphasizing that inclusion must extend beyond normative ideals into institutional implementation. Islamic ethics demands that values such as justice (*ʿadl*), mercy (*raḥmah*), and trust (*amānah*) be operationalized within curriculum design, pedagogical strategies, and school governance (Kamali, 2022a, 2022b). Inclusion, therefore, requires proactive efforts to identify and dismantle physical, curricular, and attitudinal barriers that hinder participation. Contemporary scholarship in Islamic education highlights that ethical commitments gain meaning only when translated into sustained practice (Auda, 2021). From this perspective, inclusive education becomes a moral obligation expressed through deliberate structural and pedagogical reform.

Teachers occupy a central role in translating Islamic moral values into inclusive classroom practice. Within Islamic ethical thought, educators function as moral agents (*fāʿil akhlāqī*), whose beliefs and attitudes toward disability significantly influence learners' experiences (Ghaly, 2022). Inclusive outcomes are shaped not only by technical competence but also by teachers' moral sensitivity, empathy, and reflective practice. Teacher education programs in Muslim contexts must therefore integrate ethical formation alongside pedagogical training. When teachers embody Islamic values of compassion and justice, inclusion becomes an enacted ethic rather than a procedural requirement, fostering learning environments that affirm dignity and participation for all students.

Institutional commitment is equally essential and reflects the Qurʾānic principle of *amānah* (trust). Educational authorities and school leaders are entrusted with safeguarding learners' rights and ensuring equitable access to quality education (Kamali, 2022a, 2022b). Policies that neglect accessibility, teacher support, or inclusive infrastructure represent a breach of this trust. Islamic governance ethics frame leadership as moral stewardship, requiring accountability to both society and God. Consequently, institutional inclusion is not merely administrative compliance but a manifestation of ethical responsibility. Schools and universities function as collective moral actors whose structures either enable or obstruct the realization of inclusive values.

By grounding inclusive education in Islamic moral theology, this chapter establishes a robust ethical foundation that resonates with both religious tradition and contemporary educational theory. Inclusion is affirmed not as a borrowed or externally imposed concept but as an authentic expression of Islam's moral vision of human dignity and social responsibility (Auda, 2021). Framing inclusion as *ʿibādah ijtimāʿiyyah* (collective worship) integrates faith with professional practice, elevating educational work to moral significance. This synthesis demonstrates that inclusive education in Muslim societies is not only pedagogically sound but theologically grounded, reinforcing its legitimacy and sustainability.

To synthesize the preceding ethical discussion into an integrated conceptual framework, Fig. 1.1 presents a logic model of Islamic ethics-based inclusive

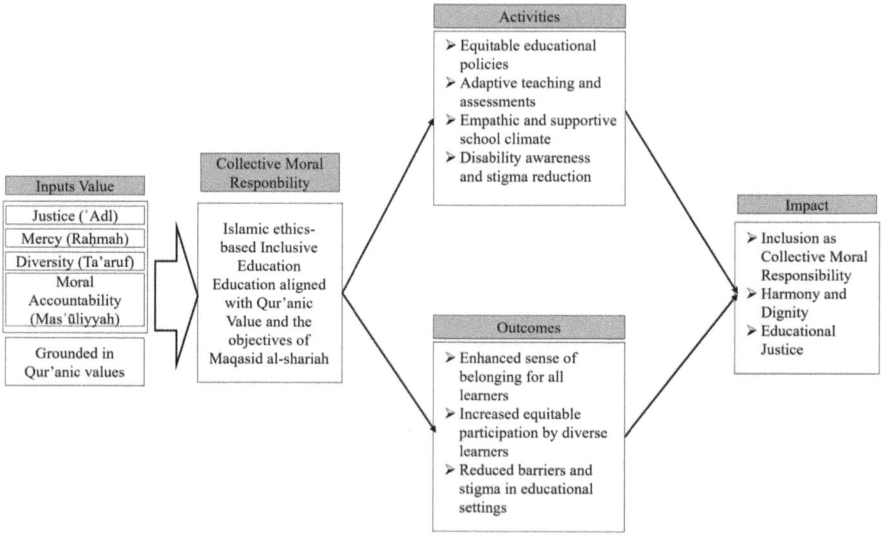

Fig. 1.1 Logic model of Islamic ethics-based inclusive education

education. The model illustrates how core Qurʾānic values justice (ʿadl), mercy (raḥmah), recognition of diversity (taʿāruf), and moral accountability (masʾūliyyah) function as foundational inputs that inform inclusive educational practices and institutional activities. These practices generate supportive learning environments and equitable participation for diverse learners, leading to inclusive educational outcomes and long-term ethical impact. Within this framework, inclusion is conceptualized not as a peripheral policy adaptation but as a form of collective moral responsibility aligned with Islamic ethical theology and the objectives of maqāṣid al-sharīʿah.

By positioning inclusion within an Islamic ethical logic model, this chapter underscores that inclusive education is inseparable from broader questions of moral agency, institutional responsibility, and social trust. Inclusion, in this sense, is not limited to pedagogical technique or administrative adjustment, but reflects how educational institutions embody ethical commitments in everyday practice. The framework invites educators and policymakers to move beyond compliance-driven approaches and to critically examine whose needs are prioritized, whose voices are recognized, and how power operates within educational spaces. Framing inclusion as an ethical orientation rooted in Islamic moral theology strengthens its normative legitimacy while opening space for contextualized implementation across diverse Muslim educational settings.

1.9 Conclusion

This chapter has demonstrated that inclusive education can be coherently and normatively grounded within Islamic moral theology rather than treated as an externally derived or purely policy-driven construct. Through an analysis of Qurʾānic principles, such as human dignity (*karāmah al-insān*), justice (*ʿadl*), mercy (*raḥmah*), diversity (*taʿāruf*), and moral accountability (*masʾūliyyah*), the chapter has articulated an ethical framework that affirms the full moral status of learners with disabilities. When situated within the objectives of Islamic law (*maqāṣid al-sharīʿah*), inclusion emerges as a central ethical and legal imperative aimed at protecting intellect, life, and honor. This framework challenges deficit-based narratives and reframes disability as part of divinely intended human diversity rather than deviation or deficiency. By bridging Islamic moral theology with educational praxis, this chapter contributes to both Islamic educational scholarship and contemporary inclusive education theory. Conceptualizing inclusion as *ʿibādah ijtimāʿiyyah* (collective moral responsibility) integrates faith-based ethics with professional and institutional accountability. This approach enhances the cultural and ethical legitimacy of inclusive education in Muslim contexts while remaining compatible with global inclusion frameworks that emphasize equity, participation, and belonging. Future research may extend this framework through empirical studies, policy analysis, and teacher education models informed by Islamic ethics. Ultimately, grounding inclusion in Islamic moral vision offers a sustainable and internally coherent pathway toward educational systems that honor dignity, justice, and meaningful participation for all learners.

References

Abou El Fadl, K. (2022). *Reasoning with God: Reclaiming Shariʻah in the modern age*. Rowman & Littlefield.

Auda, J. (2021). *Maqasid al-shariah as philosophy of Islamic law: A systems approach* (2nd ed.). International Institute of Islamic Thought.

Bazna, M. S., & Hatab, T. A. (2020). Disability in Islam: A moral framework for inclusive education. *Journal of Religion, Disability & Health, 24*(3), 287–302. https://doi.org/10.1080/15228967.2020.1779672

Bazna, M., & Hatab, T. A. (2022). *Disability in the Islamic tradition: Ethics, jurisprudence, and inclusion*. Routledge.

Florian, L. (2019). On the necessary co-existence of special and inclusive education. *International Journal of Inclusive Education, 23*(7–8), 691–704. https://doi.org/10.1080/13603116.2019.1622801

Ghaly, M. (2019). *Islamic bioethics in the twenty-first century*. Routledge.

Ghaly, M. (2022). *Islamic ethics and disability: Justice, dignity, and moral responsibility*. Routledge.

Hallaq, W. B. (2019). *Reforming modernity: Ethics and the new humanism in Islam*. Columbia University Press.

Kamali, M. H. (2021a). *Human dignity in Islam: Foundations and implications*. International Institute of Islamic Thought.
Kamali, M. H. (2021b). *Human dignity, justice, and rights in Islam*. International Institute of Islamic Thought.
Kamali, M. H. (2022a). *The ethical foundations of Islam*. International Institute of Islamic Thought.
Kamali, M. H. (2022b). *The Islamic ethics of compassion and mercy*. International Institute of Islamic Thought.
Saeed, A. (2020). *Interpreting the Qur'an: Towards a contemporary approach*. Routledge.
Slee, R. (2023). *Inclusive education isn't dead, it just smells funny* (2nd ed.). Routledge.
UNESCO. (2020). *Global education monitoring report 2020: Inclusion and education - All means all*. UNESCO.
United Nations. (2016). *Convention on the rights of persons with disabilities*. United Nations.

Chapter 2
Confronting Social Attitudes and Stigma

Abstract This chapter critically examines social attitudes and stigma surrounding disability in Muslim societies, with particular attention to education and employment contexts. Drawing on Islamic ethical principles and contemporary disability studies, the chapter argues that stigma is not rooted in Islamic theology but is sustained through culturally embedded beliefs, institutional norms, and structural inequalities. Using Indonesia as a contextual case, the analysis highlights the persistent gap between public endorsement of disability rights and everyday practices that marginalize persons with disabilities. The chapter explores how ableist assumptions are reproduced through family decision-making, educational systems, and labor markets, despite strong theological commitments to human dignity, justice, and compassion. By framing stigma as a form of structural injustice and ethical failure, the chapter advances an integrative framework that bridges Islamic moral theology with inclusive education and social policy. This ethical analysis provides a foundation for reorienting institutions toward equity, participation, and moral accountability within Muslim societies.

Keywords Disability Stigma · Islamic Ethics · Inclusive Education · Human Dignity · Social Justice

2.1 Introduction

Despite significant advances in disability rights discourse within Muslim societies, social stigma toward persons with disabilities remains deeply entrenched. Legal reforms, inclusive education policies, and religious affirmations of compassion have not fully translated into everyday social inclusion. In many contexts, disability continues to be framed through cultural narratives of deficiency, moral failing, or dependency, shaping how individuals and institutions respond to difference (Bazna & Hatab, 2020; Shakespeare, 2018). This chapter argues that stigma is not merely attitudinal but structural, sustained by social norms, institutional arrangements, and

K. Bashori, Z. Nuryana, *Disability Inclusion*, SpringerBriefs in Modern Perspectives on Disability Research,
https://doi.org/10.1007/978-981-95-8907-4_2

unexamined assumptions. Understanding how stigma operates within Muslim communities is therefore essential for bridging the gap between ethical ideals and lived realities, particularly in educational and employment contexts where exclusion remains most pronounced.

Islamic theology offers robust ethical resources that affirm human dignity (*karāmah al-insān*), justice (*ʿadl*), and compassion (*raḥmah*) as universal moral imperatives. Qurʾānic teachings and Prophetic practice consistently reject any association between bodily difference and spiritual inferiority. However, these normative theological principles often coexist with social practices that marginalize persons with disabilities through pity, avoidance, or paternalism (Ghaly, 2022). This tension between theology and practice highlights the sociocultural mediation of religious ethics. Rather than being driven by doctrine, stigma is frequently produced through cultural interpretation, institutional inertia, and power relations. Examining this dissonance allows for a more precise diagnosis of why exclusion persists despite strong religious commitments to inclusion.

The Indonesian context provides a particularly instructive case for analyzing this tension. Indonesia has ratified international disability rights and conventions and enacted progressive national legislation supporting inclusion. Public discourse increasingly reflects support for disability rights, inclusive education, and workplace diversity (Tamba, 2017; United Nations, 2006). Yet, empirical studies reveal persistent gaps between policy and practice, as families, schools, and employers continue to make exclusionary decisions (Kurniawati et al., 2022; Sunardi et al., 2021). These contradictions illustrate how stigma operates subtly through fear, risk aversion, and normative expectations rather than overt discrimination. Situating this analysis within Indonesia enables a grounded exploration of how global rights frameworks intersect with local religious and cultural dynamics.

This chapter therefore examines stigma as a form of structural injustice and ethical failure rather than an individual moral flaw. By integrating Islamic ethical analysis with contemporary disability studies and empirical research, the chapter moves beyond descriptive accounts of stigma toward a critical moral evaluation. Educational and employment systems are analyzed as key sites where ableist norms are reproduced and legitimated. The chapter argues that addressing stigma requires ethical reorientation, institutional accountability, and cultural critique grounded in Islamic moral philosophy and human rights principles (Kamali, 2021; WHO, 2023). This approach lays the foundation for subsequent chapters that focus on ethical frameworks and practical strategies for advancing inclusive education in Muslim societies.

2.2 Disability as Curse or Divine Punishment: Cultural Interpretive Frameworks

In many Muslim communities, disability continues to be interpreted through cultural frameworks that associate imlErment with divine punishment, curse, or ancestral wrongdoing. These interpretations are often shaped by local traditions, syncretic belief systems, and informal religious narratives rather than by rigorous engagement with *Qurʾānic* theology (Bazna & Hatab, 2020). In Indonesia, disability beliefs frequently intersect with pre-Islamic cosmologies, spiritual folklore, and communal myths that moralize bodily difference. Disability is thus framed not as a neutral human condition but as a sign requiring moral explanation. Such interpretations persist through oral transmission and everyday discourse, shaping social attitudes long before formal religious education intervenes. As a result, stigma becomes embedded within cultural common sense rather than openly articulated theological doctrine.

The moralization of disability has significant social consequences, particularly in relation to shame (*hayāʾ*) and collective reputation. Families may experience disability as a source of social anxiety, fearing judgment from neighbors, religious peers, or extended kin networks. Consequently, children and adults with disabilities are sometimes hidden from public view, excluded from social gatherings, or discouraged from participating in communal life (Al-Aoufi et al., 2012). Educational enrollment may be delayed, and access to health or support services limited, not due to lack of awareness but due to fear of stigma. These practices reinforce social invisibility and normalize exclusion as a protective strategy. Stigma thus operates not only at the level of belief but through everyday family decisions shaped by communal expectations.

Islamic theology, however, offers a fundamentally different interpretive framework for understanding disability. The Qurʾān repeatedly emphasizes that trials (*balāʾ*) are universal, ethically neutral, and distributed without regard to moral worth (Ghaly, 2022). Physical imIErment is not presented as evidence of divine displeasure nor is bodily normalcy equated with spiritual superiority. Classical Islamic scholars caution against linking suffering to sin, emphasizing humility in interpreting divine will. Despite this theological clarity, cultural interpretations often overshadow doctrinal teachings in everyday life. This disjunction illustrates how religious concepts can be selectively appropriated or distorted through cultural lenses, allowing stigma to persist under the appearance of religious legitimacy.

The persistence of these cultural interpretive frameworks reflects a broader gap between normative Islamic doctrine and lived religious culture. Disability-related stigma is sustained not by explicit theological endorsement but by unexamined cultural assumptions that become religiously coded over time (Saeed, 2020). Such assumptions legitimize exclusion while remaining largely invisible as ethical problems. From an Islamic ethical perspective, this represents a failure of moral reflection rather than a limitation of theology. Addressing disability stigma therefore requires critical engagement with cultural narratives alongside theological education. By disentangling Islamic ethics from inherited cultural interpretations, Muslim communities can challenge stigma and reframe disability as part of divinely intended human diversity.

2.3 Theological Teachings of Compassion and Human Dignity

Islamic ethics firmly ground social relations in compassion (*raḥmah*), justice (*ʿadl*), and human dignity (*karāmah al-insān*), which function as foundational moral principles in the *Qurʾān* and Prophetic tradition. Numerous Qurʾānic passages affirm the inherent worth of all human beings by virtue of their creation, irrespective of physical or cognitive ability (Qurʾān 17:70). Contemporary Islamic scholarship emphasizes that dignity is ontological and unconditional, not contingent upon bodily normalcy or social productivity (Kamali, 2021). Prophetic practices further reinforce this view through inclusive engagement with individuals of varying abilities. Within this ethical framework, persons with disabilities are recognized as full moral agents (*mukallaf*), equally accountable and equally honored before God, thereby rejecting any theological basis for marginalization or hierarchy.

Despite the clarity of these ethical principles, their translation into everyday social practice remains limited. Religious discourse in many Muslim communities frequently emphasizes compassion in the form of charity (*ṣadaqah*) and benevolence, framing disability primarily as an object of care rather than a subject of rights (Bazna & Hatab, 2020). While such practices reflect goodwill, they often fail to challenge deeper patterns of exclusion embedded within educational, economic, and social institutions. Mercy becomes individualized and episodic rather than structural and transformative. As a result, persons with disabilities may be cared for but not included, supported but not empowered, revealing a gap between ethical ideals and lived realities.

This disconnection reflects a broader tendency to interpret compassion narrowly, as emotional kindness rather than ethical responsibility. Islamic moral philosophy, however, understands *raḥmah* as an active moral commitment that demands justice, inclusion, and protection from harm (Ghaly, 2022). Compassion, in this sense, requires addressing the conditions that restrict participation and reinforce dependency. When Islamic ethics is reduced to charitable sentiment, it risks reinforcing paternalism and masking structural injustice. A rights-affirming interpretation of compassion therefore calls for ethical engagement with accessibility, equity, and institutional accountability, particularly in education and employment contexts where exclusion remains prevalent.

Moving beyond symbolic compassion requires reinterpreting Islamic ethical teachings through a justice-oriented and rights-based lens. Affirming human dignity (*karāmah*) entails recognizing agency, voice, and participation as essential components of ethical inclusion (Kamali, 2021). Persons with disabilities must be engaged not merely as recipients of mercy but as active contributors to communal life. Such an approach aligns Islamic theology with contemporary inclusive education frameworks that emphasize belonging and participation. By bridging compassion with justice, Islamic ethics provides a powerful moral foundation for transforming social practices and addressing structural exclusion, ensuring that theological commitments are realized in everyday institutional and communal contexts.

2.4 The Tension Between Normative Theology and Lived Social Practice

A central challenge in disability inclusion within Muslim societies lies in the tension between normative Islamic theology and lived social practice. Islamic teachings explicitly affirm inclusion, equality, and respect for all human beings, grounding these values in concepts of dignity (*karāmah*), justice (*ʿadl*), and compassion (*raḥmah*). However, everyday social interactions often reflect avoidance, pity, or paternalistic attitudes toward persons with disabilities (Bazna & Hatab, 2020). This dissonance indicates that stigma is not rooted in theological doctrine but in sociocultural norms that shape behavior more powerfully than abstract ethical commitments. As a result, religious values may be verbally endorsed while remaining insufficiently embodied in daily practices, allowing exclusion to persist without being perceived as an ethical contradiction.

The persistence of stigma despite strong theological resources highlights the selective appropriation of religious teachings. In many contexts, Islamic ethics are invoked symbolically to promote charity and compassion, while more demanding ethical implications such as rights, accessibility, and institutional reform are overlooked (Ghaly, 2022). This selective application allows discriminatory practices to coexist with religious piety, as exclusion is framed as a social or practical issue rather than a moral failing. Individuals and institutions may thus perceive themselves as ethically compliant while perpetuating marginalization. This dynamic underscores the need to distinguish between normative theology and its social enactment, particularly in relation to disability inclusion.

Sociological studies in Indonesia further illustrate how cultural norms mediate religious interpretation in everyday life. Community expectations regarding normalcy, productivity, and social harmony often override theological commitments to inclusion, shaping how disability is perceived and managed (Saeed, 2020). Pity and overprotection, though seemingly benevolent, function as mechanisms of control that limit autonomy and participation. Such practices are rarely recognized as discriminatory because they are culturally normalized and morally justified through selective readings of compassion. Consequently, stigma operates subtly through social routines and institutional habits rather than explicit exclusion or hostility.

Understanding the tension between normative theology and lived practice is essential for developing effective inclusion strategies in Muslim societies. Without addressing the sociocultural filters through which theology is interpreted, ethical teachings risk remaining abstract and disconnected from institutional realities. Bridging this gap requires critical ethical reflection, religious education, and structural reform that align social practice with theological commitments (Kamali, 2021). By foregrounding this tension, Islamic ethics can be mobilized not merely as symbolic rhetoric but as a transformative moral force capable of challenging stigma and fostering genuine inclusion in education, employment, and community life.

2.5 Public Endorsement of Disability Rights and Private Resistance

Recent developments in Indonesia indicate increasing public endorsement of disability rights, influenced by national legislation, international conventions, and religious advocacy. The ratification of the Convention on the Rights of Persons with Disabilities (CRPD) and the enactment of Law No. 8/2016 have strengthened public discourse around inclusion, accessibility, and equality (United Nations, 2006; Tamba, 2017). Religious leaders and organizations have also issued statements emphasizing compassion and dignity for persons with disabilities. However, this formal endorsement often remains at the level of rhetoric, functioning as symbolic compliance rather than transformative commitment. While inclusion is publicly affirmed as a moral and legal ideal, its practical implications are frequently resisted in everyday social contexts.

This contradiction is especially evident in family decision-making processes. Parents may express agreement with inclusive education policies while privately discouraging school attendance for children with disabilities due to fear of bullying, academic failure, or social stigma (Kurniawati et al., 2022). Such decisions are often framed as protective rather than exclusionary, masking underlying assumptions about limited capability and social risk. Cultural expectations surrounding normality, achievement, and family reputation further shape these choices. As a result, inclusion is supported in principle but constrained in practice, revealing how stigma operates through affective concerns and moral ambivalence rather than overt rejection.

Educational institutions similarly display a gap between inclusive discourse and institutional behavior. Schools may adopt inclusive terminology in mission statements and policy documents while resisting curricular adaptation, teacher training, or resource allocation necessary for meaningful inclusion (Sunardi et al., 2021). Inclusion is frequently treated as an administrative requirement rather than a pedagogical transformation. Teachers may express support for students with disabilities yet feel unprepared or unwilling to modify assessment practices or classroom routines. This form of institutional resistance reflects risk aversion and performance-oriented cultures that prioritize standardization over equity, thereby reproducing exclusion within ostensibly inclusive frameworks.

In employment contexts, private resistance becomes particularly visible despite widespread public support for diversity. Employers may endorse disability inclusion rhetorically while avoiding the recruitment or retention of persons with disabilities due to perceived costs, productivity concerns, or workplace disruption (ILO, 2022). These attitudes are rarely articulated as discrimination but justified through managerial pragmatism and economic rationality. Such practices demonstrate how stigma persists through unexamined assumptions rather than explicit bias. Addressing this gap requires not only legal enforcement but cultural and ethical transformation that aligns private decision-making with publicly endorsed commitments to disability rights.

2.6 Educational Exclusion and Ableist Institutional Norms

Educational institutions constitute a central arena in which social stigma toward disability becomes formalized and reproduced through policy and practice. Standardized curricula, norm-referenced assessments, and rigid pacing structures often privilege a narrow conception of ability, implicitly marginalizing learners who diverge from these norms. Such systems are grounded in ableist assumptions that equate intelligence with speed, independence, and uniform performance (Hehir, 2020). As a result, students with disabilities are frequently positioned as deficient rather than differently abled. These institutional norms shape expectations, influence teacher attitudes, and limit opportunities for meaningful participation. Educational exclusion, therefore, emerges not as an individual failure but as a systemic outcome of structures that prioritize conformity over equity.

In the Indonesian context, inclusive education has been formally endorsed through national policy and legislative frameworks. However, implementation remains uneven due to limited resources, insufficient teacher preparation, and inconsistent institutional commitment (Sunardi et al., 2021). Many schools lack accessible infrastructure, assistive technologies, and specialized support personnel. Teachers often report uncertainty in adapting curricula and assessments for diverse learners, leading to reliance on exclusionary practices such as tracking or informal segregation. Cultural beliefs that associate disability with incapacity further exacerbate these challenges. Consequently, inclusion is frequently interpreted as physical placement rather than pedagogical transformation, reinforcing ableist norms within ostensibly inclusive environments.

Assessment practices play a particularly significant role in sustaining educational exclusion. High-stakes testing and uniform evaluation criteria often fail to account for diverse learning profiles, disproportionately disadvantaging students with disabilities (Ainscow, 2020). When academic success is narrowly defined, learners who require alternative modes of demonstration are perceived as underperforming or incapable. This deficit-oriented framework not only limits educational attainment but also contributes to internalized stigma and reduced self-efficacy. Islamic educational ethics challenge such practices by emphasizing the cultivation of intellect according to individual capacity rather than standardized benchmarks. Failure to accommodate diversity in assessment thus represents both a pedagogical and moral shortcoming.

From an Islamic ethical perspective, educational exclusion contradicts the obligation to protect intellect (*ḥifẓ al-ʿaql*) and uphold human dignity (*karāmah al-insān*). Knowledge is regarded as a trust (amānah) that must be made accessible to all learners, regardless of ability (Kamali, 2019). Institutional practices that systematically disadvantage students with disabilities constitute a form of injustice (*ẓulm*), even when unintentional. Addressing educational exclusion therefore requires more than technical reform; it necessitates ethical reflection and institutional accountability. Inclusive education, when grounded in Islamic values, becomes a moral imperative aimed at restoring equity, dignity, and intellectual flourishing for all learners.

2.7 Employment, Productivity, and Social Worth

Employment practices constitute a significant domain in which disability-related stigma is reproduced through assumptions about productivity, independence, and economic value. In many Muslim societies, including Indonesia, social worth is often implicitly linked to one's capacity for IEd labor and self-sufficiency (ILO, 2022). Persons with disabilities are frequently perceived as dependent, inefficient, or costly, reinforcing their marginalization in formal labor markets. These perceptions persist despite legal protections and policy commitments to workplace inclusion. As a result, exclusion from employment is normalized through economic rationalizations rather than recognized as a form of discrimination, thereby obscuring its ethical implications.

Legal frameworks supporting employment inclusion have expanded in recent years, yet their implementation remains limited. Employers may publicly endorse disability inclusion while privately resisting reasonable accommodations due to concerns about cost, productivity, or workplace disruption (Schur et al., 2021). Normative productivity standards privilege speed, uniform performance, and uninterrupted availability, disadvantaging workers with disabilities whose contributions may take alternative forms. Such standards reflect ableist labor cultures rather than objective measures of competence. Consequently, inclusion initiatives often focus on compliance rather than meaningful participation, leaving structural barriers intact and reinforcing employment exclusion.

Islamic ethical thought fundamentally challenges the reduction of human value to economic output. While work is encouraged as a means of personal fulfillment and social contribution, dignity (*karāmah*) is understood as inherent and not contingent upon productivity (Kamali, 2019). Islamic jurisprudence emphasizes social responsibility (*takāful ijtimāʿī*) and mutual support, recognizing that human capacities vary by divine design. From this perspective, excluding individuals from employment solely on the basis of disability constitutes a form of injustice (*ẓulm*) that violates ethical obligations toward equity and compassion. Employment, therefore, should be structured to accommodate diversity rather than enforce uniformity.

Addressing employment exclusion requires both ethical reorientation and institutional reform. Inclusive labor practices must challenge dominant productivity narratives and recognize diverse forms of contribution, including relational, cognitive, and experiential labor (WHO, 2023). Policies promoting workplace accessibility, flexible arrangements, and reasonable accommodations should be framed not as charity but as ethical and social obligations. Within an Islamic framework, enabling meaningful participation in work aligns with the pursuit of social justice and collective well-being (*maṣlaḥah*). Reframing employment inclusion as a moral responsibility rather than an economic concession is essential for dismantling stigma and advancing social equity.

2.8 Stigma as Structural Injustice and Ethical Failure

Stigma surrounding disability should be understood not merely as an individual attitude but as a form of structural injustice embedded within social systems, institutional practices, and cultural norms. Educational, economic, and religious institutions often privilege able-bodied standards while marginalizing or rendering disability invisible (Shakespeare, 2018). These structural dynamics shape opportunities, distribute resources unevenly, and normalize exclusion without requiring explicit discriminatory intent. As a result, stigma becomes self-reinforcing, operating through policies, procedures, and expectations that systematically disadvantage persons with disabilities. Recognizing stigma as structural shifts the focus from moral blame toward ethical responsibility, highlighting the need for systemic transformation rather than isolated interventions.

Institutional arrangements play a decisive role in sustaining disability-related stigma. When schools, workplaces, and public spaces are designed around able-bodied norms, exclusion is framed as an individual limitation rather than a structural failure (Ainscow, 2020). Such environments implicitly communicate who belongs and who does not, shaping social hierarchies and internalized identities. These dynamics are further reinforced by power relations that marginalize disabled voices in decision-making processes. Consequently, stigma persists not because of overt hostility but due to institutional inertia and unexamined assumptions embedded within organizational cultures and governance structures.

From an Islamic ethical perspective, structural stigma constitutes a collective moral failure rather than a series of isolated ethical lapses. Islamic moral philosophy emphasizes responsibility (*masʾūliyyah*) not only at the individual level but also at the institutional and societal levels (Kamali, 2019). Institutions entrusted with education, employment, and public welfare bear an ethical obligation to ensure equitable participation and prevent harm. When exclusionary structures persist, they represent a form of injustice (*ẓulm*) that contradicts Qurʾānic imperatives of justice (*ʿadl*) and compassion (*raḥmah*). Ethical accountability, therefore, extends beyond personal intentions to encompass systemic outcomes.

Addressing stigma as structural injustice requires a multidimensional ethical response. Attitudinal change alone is insufficient without accompanying policy reform, institutional redesign, and mechanisms of accountability (WHO, 2023). Inclusion must be framed as a moral corrective project aimed at restoring dignity (karāmah), justice, and social balance. Within Muslim societies, this entails aligning institutional practices with Islamic ethical principles and contemporary human rights frameworks. By conceptualizing inclusion as an ethical obligation rather than discretionary benevolence, stigma can be dismantled at its structural roots, enabling more just and participatory social arrangements.

2.9 Conclusion

This chapter has demonstrated that disability-related stigma in Muslim societies is sustained less by Islamic theology than by culturally embedded interpretations, institutional practices, and structural norms. Despite strong theological foundations affirming human dignity, justice, and compassion, stigma persists through moralized beliefs, ableist educational systems, and exclusionary employment practices. The analysis reveals a persistent gap between normative Islamic ethics and lived social realities, where inclusion is often endorsed rhetorically but resisted in practice. By framing stigma as a structural injustice rather than an individual prejudice, this chapter highlights the ethical responsibility of institutions and communities to address exclusion as a collective moral failure. Importantly, the chapter positions Islamic ethics as a critical resource for transformative inclusion rather than symbolic accommodation. Concepts such as *karāmah al-insān*, *ʿadl*, *raḥmah*, and *maqāṣid al-sharīʿah* provide a robust moral framework for challenging ableist norms and reorienting educational and social institutions toward equity and participation. Addressing stigma therefore requires ethical reorientation alongside policy reform, institutional accountability, and cultural critique. When inclusion is understood as a moral imperative grounded in Islamic values and aligned with contemporary human rights frameworks, it becomes a corrective project aimed at restoring dignity, justice, and social balance within Muslim societies.

References

Ainscow, M. (2020). Promoting inclusion and equity in education: Lessons from international experiences. *Nordic Journal of Studies in Educational Policy, 6*(1), 7–16. https://doi.org/10.1080/20020317.2020.1729587

Al-Aoufi, H., Al-Zyoud, N., & Shahminan, N. (2012). Islam and the cultural conceptualisation of disability. *International Journal of Adolescence and Youth, 17*(4), 205–219. https://doi.org/10.1080/02673843.2011.649565

Bazna, M. S., & Hatab, T. A. (2020). Disability in Islam: A moral framework for inclusive education. *Journal of Religion, Disability & Health, 24*(3), 287–302. https://doi.org/10.1080/15228967.2020.1779672

Ghaly, M. (2022). *Islamic ethics and disability: Justice, dignity, and moral responsibility*. Routledge.

Hehir, T. (2020). *Ableism in education: Rethinking school practices and policies*. Harvard Education Press.

International Labour Organization. (2022). *Disability inclusion in the workplace: Policy and practice*. ILO.

Kamali, M. H. (2019). *The middle path of moderation in Islam: The Qurʾānic principle of wasaity. or*. Oxford University Press.

Kamali, M. H. (2021). *Human dignity, justice, and rights in Islam*. International Institute of Islamic Thought.

Kurniawati, F., Minnaert, A., Mangunsong, F., & Ahmed, W. (2022). Parental beliefs and inclusive education in Indonesia. *International Journal of Inclusive Education, 26*(10), 1045–1061. https://doi.org/10.1080/13603116.2020.1713744

Saeed, A. (2020). *Interpreting the Qur'an: Towards a contemporary approach.* Routledge.

Schur, L., Ameri, M., & Kruse, D. (2021). Telework after COVID: A "silver lining" for workers with disabilities? *Journal of Occupational Rehabilitation, 31*(3), 521–536. https://doi.org/10.1007/s10926-021-09936-5

Shakespeare, T. (2018). *Disability: The basics*. Routledge.

Sunardi, M. Y., Gunarhadi, P., & Yeager, J. L. (2021). Inclusive education in Indonesia: Policy, practice, and challenges. *International Journal of Disability, Development and Education, 68*(1), 1–18. https://doi.org/10.1080/1034912X.2019.1703720

Tamba, J. (2017). A juridical study toward Indonesian disabilities right for public services accessibility according to law no. 8 year 2016. *IJDS: Indonesian Journal of Disability Studies, 4*(1), 63–68. https://doi.org/10.21776/ub.ijds.2017.004.01.9

United Nations. (2006). *Convention on the rights of persons with disabilities*. UN.

World Health Organization. (2023). *Global report on health equity for persons with disabilities*. WHO.

Chapter 3
Curriculum Adaptation and Pedagogy in Islamic Education

Abstract This chapter examines curriculum adaptation and pedagogical strategies for inclusive Islamic Religious Education (*Pendidikan Agama Islam*, IE), with a focus on accommodating learners with disabilities in Muslim school contexts. Drawing on Islamic ethical principles and contemporary inclusive education theory, the chapter argues that meaningful inclusion in IE requires adaptive curriculum design, learner-centered pedagogy, and ethical institutional commitment. Through analysis of practices in Indonesian inclusive schools, the chapter highlights the use of multisensory instruction, differentiated learning, Individualized Education Programs (IEPs), and inclusive assessment to enhance participation and spiritual engagement. The findings demonstrate that adaptive pedagogies not only improve learning outcomes but also affirm human dignity, justice, and mercy as core Islamic values. By integrating moral theology with classroom practice, the chapter positions inclusive IE as both a pedagogical innovation and an ethical enactment of Islamic educational philosophy.

Keywords Inclusive Education · Islamic Religious Education · Curriculum Adaptation · Differentiated Instruction · Disability Inclusion (Indonesia)

3.1 Introduction

Inclusive education has increasingly been recognized as a global ethical and pedagogical imperative, yet its practical realization within faith-based educational systems requires careful contextualization. In Islamic education, inclusion must be articulated not only through policy discourse but through curriculum design and pedagogical practice that resonate with Islamic moral philosophy. This chapter addresses the intersection between inclusive education and Islamic Religious Education (*Pendidikan Agama Islam*, IE), arguing that meaningful inclusion depends on adaptive pedagogies that honor learner diversity while preserving theological integrity. Recent scholarship emphasizes that inclusive education is most

K. Bashori, Z. Nuryana, *Disability Inclusion*, SpringerBriefs in Modern Perspectives on Disability Research,
https://doi.org/10.1007/978-981-95-8907-4_3

sustainable when grounded in locally relevant ethical frameworks rather than imported models alone (Ainscow, 2020; UNESCO, 2020).

Islamic Religious Education occupies a distinctive position within Muslim schooling as a compulsory subject responsible for transmitting religious knowledge, ethical values, and spiritual orientation. Consequently, exclusion within IE carries profound moral implications, as it risks marginalizing learners from religious meaning-making and communal belonging. Drawing on Islamic ethical principles, such as human dignity (*karāmah*), justice (*ʿadl*), mercy (*raḥmah*), and capacity (*istiṭāʿah*), this chapter conceptualizes curriculum adaptation as a moral responsibility rather than a pedagogical concession (Kamali, 2021; Bazna & Hatab, 2020). Disability, from this perspective, is not an obstacle to religious learning but an expression of human diversity that demands responsive instructional design.

This chapter situates its analysis within the Indonesian educational context, where inclusive education policies coexist with significant challenges in implementation. While national regulations promote inclusive schooling, Islamic Religious Education often remains characterized by standardized curricula, text-centered instruction, and uniform assessment practices that disadvantage learners with disabilities (Sunardi et al., 2021). Through engagement with empirical studies and school-based practices, this chapter highlights how curriculum adaptation, multisensory instruction, differentiated learning, and Individualized Education Programs (IEPs) are being applied within inclusive Islamic schools. These practices demonstrate that pedagogical flexibility can enhance engagement, reduce anxiety, and foster spiritual participation without compromising religious authenticity.

By integrating contemporary inclusive education theory with Islamic educational ethics, this chapter bridges normative ideals and classroom praxis. It positions teachers as ethical agents and institutions as moral communities entrusted with safeguarding learners' rights and dignity. The chapter argues that inclusive pedagogy in IE is not merely a technical innovation but an enactment of Islamic moral vision within educational practice. Through curriculum adaptation and learner-centered pedagogy, Islamic education can model the very values it seeks to inculcate: justice, compassion, and respect for human diversity thus contributing to more equitable and humane educational environments (Florian & Black-Hawkins, 2019; Hehir, 2020).

3.2 Inclusive Pedagogy in Islamic Education: Conceptual Foundations

Islamic Education (*Pendidikan Agama Islam*, IE) plays a foundational role in shaping learners' moral, spiritual, and social identities within Muslim schooling. As a compulsory subject, IE carries the responsibility of transmitting religious knowledge while cultivating ethical sensibilities and communal values. An inclusive pedagogical approach requires reconceptualizing IE not merely as content delivery but as a relational and ethical practice that affirms learner diversity (Ainscow, 2020). Inclusive pedagogy emphasizes equitable access to meaning-making, ensuring that all students, including those with disabilities, can engage with religious learning in ways that are cognitively, emotionally, and spiritually meaningful.

Grounded in Islamic ethics, inclusive pedagogy draws upon the principles of human dignity (*karāmah*), justice (*ʿadl*), and mercy (*raḥmah*). The Qurʾān affirms the inherent worth of all human beings irrespective of physical or cognitive differences (Qurʾān 17:70), while Prophetic pedagogy demonstrates attentiveness to individual capacity. Contemporary Islamic scholars argue that diversity in ability reflects divine intentionality rather than deficiency (Kamali, 2021). From this perspective, disability is not a deviation from the norm but an expression of human variation within creation. Inclusive IE therefore aligns ethical theology with pedagogical practice by affirming dignity as ontological and non-negotiable.

Inclusive pedagogy in IE challenges deficit-based educational models that position students with disabilities as lacking or incapable. Instead, it emphasizes capacity-based learning that recognizes multiple ways of knowing, understanding, and expressing religious meaning (Hehir, 2020). This approach resonates with contemporary educational theories that advocate learner-centered and constructivist pedagogies. Within Islamic education, it also reflects the principle of *istiṭāʿah* (capacity), which acknowledges that religious obligations and learning expectations must correspond to individual ability. Adaptation, therefore, is not an exception but a pedagogical responsibility rooted in ethical and theological commitments.

By integrating Islamic moral philosophy with inclusive educational theory, inclusive pedagogy in IE offers a coherent conceptual framework for curriculum and instructional adaptation. It positions teachers as ethical agents responsible for creating learning environments that honor diversity and promote participation. Such an approach ensures that religious education does not inadvertently reproduce exclusion but instead models the very values it seeks to teach (Bazna & Hatab, 2020). Inclusive IE thus becomes both a pedagogical strategy and a moral practice, aligning faith-based education with contemporary commitments to equity, inclusion, and human flourishing.

3.3 Curriculum Adaptation in IE: Principles and Design

Curriculum adaptation in Islamic Education involves intentional modification of learning objectives, content, and instructional pathways to accommodate diverse learner needs while preserving essential religious meanings. Adaptation is not a reduction of curricular rigor but a reconfiguration of access, ensuring that all students can engage meaningfully with Islamic teachings (Ainscow, 2020). In inclusive IE classrooms, curriculum design moves away from uniform progression toward flexible learning trajectories that recognize differences in cognitive processing, sensory access, and emotional readiness. This approach aligns with inclusive education principles that emphasize participation and understanding rather than standardized coverage, allowing religious learning to remain both authentic and accessible.

In practice, curriculum adaptation in IE includes flexible sequencing of topics, simplified theological language, and alternative representations of abstract religious concepts. Qurʾānic stories, for example, may be conveyed through visual narratives, dramatization, or concrete analogies that connect religious teachings to students' everyday experiences. Contextualization allows learners to grasp ethical meanings without requiring advanced linguistic or abstract reasoning skills (Tomlinson, 2017). Such strategies are particularly effective for students with intellectual or learning disabilities, as they reduce cognitive overload while preserving moral and spiritual content. Adaptation thus enhances comprehension without compromising doctrinal integrity.

Islamic jurisprudential principles provide strong ethical justification for curricular flexibility. Concepts such as *taysīr* (facilitation) and *rafʿ al-ḥaraj* (removal of hardship) emphasize that religious obligations should not impose undue difficulty (Kamali, 2019). These principles have long guided legal accommodations in worship and daily practice and are equally applicable to educational contexts. Applying them to curriculum design affirms that accessibility is a religiously grounded responsibility rather than a modern concession. Adapted curricula therefore reflect fidelity to Islamic legal ethics while responding to contemporary educational needs.

Empirical evidence from inclusive schools in Indonesia demonstrates the effectiveness of adapted IE curricula. Studies report increased student engagement, reduced learning anxiety, and improved participation among learners with disabilities when curricular flexibility is implemented (Sunardi et al., 2021). Students report a stronger sense of belonging and confidence in religious learning environments that acknowledge their capacities. These findings suggest that curriculum adaptation not only improves academic outcomes but also supports emotional and spiritual well-being. By integrating ethical principles with inclusive design, adapted IE curricula contribute to more equitable and humane Islamic education systems.

3.3.1 Multisensory Instruction in Teaching Islamic Concepts

Multisensory instructional strategies are central to inclusive Islamic education, particularly for learners with sensory, cognitive, or learning disabilities. By engaging multiple sensory channels: visual, auditory, tactile, and kinesthetic multisensory instruction enhances comprehension, attention, and memory (Meyer et al., 2020). In Islamic Religious Education (*Pendidikan Agama Islam*, IE), abstract concepts such as faith, intention, and morality become more accessible when presented through concrete and embodied experiences. Multisensory approaches shift learning from passive reception to active engagement, allowing students with diverse learning profiles to access religious knowledge meaningfully. This approach aligns with universal design for learning principles, which emphasize flexibility and accessibility in instructional design.

In teaching Qurʾānic recitation, multisensory methods include combining auditory modeling with visual text cues, color-coded *tajwīd* markings, and rhythmic repetition. For students with hearing or learning difficulties, visual representations of phonetic articulation and tactile tracing of Arabic letters support pronunciation and memorization (Al-Attas & Wan Mohd Nor, 2021). Ritual practices such as prayer (*ṣalāh*) can be taught through physical modeling, pictorial sequences, and guided movement, enabling learners to internalize both form and meaning. These strategies reduce cognitive load while reinforcing procedural memory, ensuring that religious practices are learned through embodied understanding rather than abstract instruction alone.

Multisensory instruction in IE closely reflects Prophetic pedagogical methods. The Prophet Muḥammad ﷺ frequently employed demonstration, repetition, questioning, and contextual explanation to convey religious teachings, adapting instruction to the audience's capacity (Halstead, 2004). Teaching through action and experience was central to early Islamic learning traditions, particularly in transmitting ritual knowledge. By drawing on this pedagogical heritage, multisensory instruction can be framed not as a modern innovation but as a revival of authentic Islamic educational practice. This alignment strengthens the theological legitimacy of inclusive pedagogy within Islamic education.

Empirical evidence from inclusive schools in Indonesia demonstrates the effectiveness of multisensory IE instruction. Case studies report increased student participation, improved retention of religious practices, and heightened self-confidence among learners with special needs (Sunardi et al., 2021). Students who previously struggled with verbal instruction alone show greater engagement when learning is experiential and interactive. Teachers also report more positive classroom dynamics and reduced behavioral challenges. These findings suggest that multisensory instruction transforms religious learning into an inclusive, embodied, and meaningful experience, fostering both spiritual engagement and educational equity.

3.3.2 *Differentiated Instruction and Learner-Centered IE*

Differentiated instruction in Islamic Education involves intentional variation in content, learning processes, and expected outcomes to respond to students' readiness levels, interests, and learning profiles. Rather than assuming uniform mastery, differentiated pedagogy provides multiple pathways for engaging with Islamic teachings, allowing students to access religious meaning according to their capacities (Tomlinson, 2017). This approach aligns with learner-centered education models that emphasize agency, relevance, and engagement. In inclusive IE classrooms, differentiation ensures that religious instruction remains meaningful for students with diverse cognitive, sensory, and emotional needs, thereby promoting equity without compromising core religious values.

From an Islamic ethical perspective, differentiated instruction reflects the principle of *istiṭāʿah* (capacity), which acknowledges individual variation in responsibility and obligation. Islamic jurisprudence recognizes that religious duties are contingent upon ability, reinforcing the legitimacy of pedagogical adaptation (Kamali, 2019). Applying this principle to IE affirms that learning expectations must correspond to learners' capabilities rather than standardized benchmarks. Differentiation thus becomes an ethical obligation rather than a methodological preference. By honoring individual capacity, learner-centered IE affirms students' dignity and agency, positioning them as active participants in religious learning rather than passive recipients of instruction.

Differentiation in IE can take multiple practical forms, including tiered assignments, flexible grouping, alternative tasks, and varied pacing. For example, while some students may engage in textual analysis of Qurʾānic verses, others may demonstrate understanding through storytelling, visual representation, or role-play. Such practices support collaborative learning environments where diversity is normalized and valued (Ainscow, 2020). Flexible grouping allows students to learn with and from peers, reducing social isolation and fostering mutual respect. These strategies benefit not only students with disabilities but all learners by creating inclusive classrooms that emphasize shared growth over competition.

Empirical evidence from Indonesian inclusive schools indicates that differentiated IE instruction enhances engagement, motivation, and social interaction among students with and without disabilities (Marlina et al., 2023). Teachers report improved classroom climate and increased participation when learning tasks are responsive to individual needs. Importantly, differentiation shifts the focus of assessment from performance comparison to personal growth and ethical understanding. By prioritizing process over uniform outcomes, learner-centered IE supports holistic development and reinforces the moral aims of Islamic education. Differentiated instruction thus emerges as a key strategy for fostering inclusive, ethical, and meaningful religious learning.

3.3.3 Individualized Education Programs (IEPs) in Islamic Education Instruction

Individualized Education Programs (IEPs) offer a systematic framework for aligning Islamic Religious Education (*Pendidikan Agama Islam*, IE) with students' unique abilities, needs, and learning trajectories. Within inclusive Islamic schools in Indonesia, IEPs function as pedagogical tools that translate inclusive policy into classroom practice. These individualized plans ensure that religious instruction is not limited by standardized curricula but instead reflects learner diversity. By identifying specific learning goals, instructional strategies, and assessment methods, IEPs enable students with disabilities to meaningfully engage with Islamic teachings. This approach reframes inclusion as intentional planning rather than accommodation, reinforcing the ethical imperative of equitable access to religious education (UNESCO, 2020).

The development of IEPs in IE typically involves collaborative processes among general teachers, special educators, school counselors, and parents. Such collaboration reflects shared moral responsibility (*mas'ūliyyah mushtarakah*) in supporting learners' religious development. Parental involvement is particularly significant in Islamic education, as religious learning extends beyond schools into family and community life. Research indicates that collaborative IEP planning enhances consistency, student motivation, and learning outcomes (Friend & Cook, 2019). In Indonesian contexts, this teamwork allows educators to integrate cultural sensitivity and religious values into individualized planning, ensuring that instructional adaptations remain theologically sound and socially relevant.

IEPs in Islamic Religious Instruction prioritize functional and meaningful religious competencies rather than abstract theological mastery. For students with intellectual or developmental disabilities, goals may focus on practical religious habits such as basic prayer movements, ethical conduct, or recognizing Islamic symbols. This focus aligns with Islamic jurisprudential principles that link religious obligation to capacity (*istiṭāʿah*) (Kamali, 2019). Instructional strategies may include repetition, modeling, visual supports, and routine-based learning. By emphasizing attainable religious practices, IEPs affirm students' spiritual agency and counter assumptions that disability limits religious participation or moral growth.

From an ethical standpoint, IEPs operationalize Islamic commitments to justice (*ʿadl*), trust (*amānah*), and care (*raḥmah*). Excluding learners from religious education due to standardized expectations constitutes an ethical failure rather than a pedagogical limitation. Empirical studies from inclusive Indonesian schools show that IEP-based IE instruction increases engagement, confidence, and a sense of belonging among students with disabilities (Kurniawati et al., 2022). IEPs thus function not only as educational instruments but as moral commitments, ensuring that Islamic Religious Education remains accessible, dignified, and responsive to all learners.

3.3.4 Inclusive Assessment and Evaluation in Islamic Education

Assessment in inclusive Islamic Education requires a fundamental shift from standardized, outcome-oriented testing toward authentic and formative evaluation. Traditional assessment models often privilege linguistic and cognitive abilities, thereby marginalizing students with disabilities. Inclusive assessment, by contrast, recognizes multiple forms of demonstrating religious understanding, including oral narration, practical performance of rituals, reflective dialogue, and observable ethical behavior. This approach aligns with contemporary assessment theory, which emphasizes learning as a developmental process rather than a static achievement

(Gipps, 2021). In inclusive IE classrooms, assessment functions as a tool for growth, feedback, and encouragement, ensuring that all learners can meaningfully participate in religious learning.

From an Islamic ethical perspective, inclusive assessment resonates strongly with principles that prioritize intention (*niyyah*), effort (*ijtihād*), and moral development over uniform outcomes. Prophetic traditions emphasize that actions are judged by intention, suggesting that sincere engagement holds greater value than technical perfection. Applying this ethic to educational assessment challenges rigid benchmarks that fail to account for individual capacity (*istiṭāʿah*). Flexible evaluation practices thus embody justice (*ʿadl*) by honoring learners' differing abilities without lowering moral expectations. Scholars argue that ethically grounded assessment strengthens learners' spiritual agency and prevents exclusion disguised as academic rigor (Kamali, 2019).

Empirical evidence from inclusive schools in Indonesia demonstrates that alternative assessment methods significantly reduce anxiety and enhance motivation among students with disabilities. Portfolio assessment, observational rubrics, self-reflection journals, and performance-based tasks allow learners to express religious understanding in ways aligned with their strengths. Teachers report improved engagement and more accurate insight into students' spiritual and ethical development (Kurniawati et al., 2022). These findings suggest that inclusive assessment is not only equitable but pedagogically superior, as it captures dimensions of learning often overlooked by standardized tests, particularly in moral and religious education.

Inclusive assessment in IE also reinforces the holistic aims of Islamic education, which seek to integrate cognition, behavior, emotion, and spirituality. Religious learning is understood not merely as knowledge acquisition but as internalization (*tazkiyah*) and ethical formation. Assessment practices that attend to character development, ritual consistency, and social interaction better reflect these aims. By adopting inclusive evaluation frameworks, Islamic schools affirm that religious education is accessible to all learners and that diversity in learning does not undermine, but enriches, spiritual formation. Inclusive assessment thus becomes an ethical and pedagogical necessity within Islamic education systems (UNESCO, 2020).

3.3.5 Teacher Competence, Collaboration, and Institutional Support

The effectiveness of inclusive Islamic Education is strongly influenced by teacher competence in inclusive pedagogy and disability awareness. Teachers play a central role in translating ethical commitments into classroom practice. Without adequate training in differentiated instruction, multisensory strategies, and inclusive assessment, inclusive policies remain largely symbolic. Research indicates that many Islamic education teachers feel underprepared to teach students with disabilities, particularly in religious subjects that are traditionally text-centered (Florian &

Black-Hawkins, 2019). Professional development programs that integrate Islamic ethical perspectives with inclusive educational theory are therefore essential for empowering teachers to design responsive and meaningful IE instruction.

Interprofessional collaboration is a critical component of effective inclusive IE implementation. Collaboration between IE teachers, special educators, school counselors, psychologists, and families enables holistic understanding of learners' needs and strengths. Such teamwork supports the development of Individualized Education Programs (IEPs) and ensures consistency between religious instruction and broader educational goals. Studies in Indonesian inclusive schools show that collaborative planning enhances instructional coherence and reduces teacher stress when working with students with disabilities (Kurniawati et al., 2022). From an Islamic perspective, collaboration reflects the principle of *taʿāwun* (mutual assistance), reinforcing collective responsibility for learners' spiritual and academic development.

Institutional support provides the structural foundation necessary for sustaining inclusive IE practices. Leadership commitment, inclusive school policies, accessible infrastructure, and adequate learning resources significantly shape teachers' capacity to enact inclusion. Where institutional cultures prioritize examination performance or uniform standards, inclusive efforts are often undermined. Conversely, schools that embed inclusion within their mission and governance frameworks demonstrate greater consistency and long-term impact (Ainscow, 2020). In Islamic education settings, institutional commitment signals recognition of inclusion as a moral obligation rather than an optional program, aligning organizational practice with ethical principles of justice and mercy.

Within an Islamic ethical framework, teaching is understood as an *amānah* (sacred trust) and a form of moral service (*khidmah*). Educators are accountable not only for content delivery but for nurturing the dignity and potential of every learner. Inclusive IE therefore represents an integration of professional responsibility and spiritual accountability. By fostering teacher competence, strengthening collaboration, and ensuring institutional support, inclusive IE emerges as both pedagogical practice and ethical enactment. This integration affirms that inclusion in Islamic education is not merely an innovation but an expression of compassion, justice, and collective moral responsibility (Bazna & Hatab, 2020).

3.4 Conclusion

This chapter has demonstrated that inclusive Islamic Religious Education (*Pendidikan Agama Islam*, IE) requires intentional curriculum adaptation and pedagogical transformation grounded in both Islamic ethics and contemporary inclusive education theory. Strategies such as multisensory instruction, differentiated learning, Individualized Education Programs (IEPs), and inclusive assessment practices illustrate how religious instruction can accommodate diverse learner needs without compromising theological integrity. By reframing disability as a dimension of

Sunardi, Y. M., Gunarhadi, P., & Yeager, J. L. (2021). Inclusive education in Indonesia: Policy, practice, and challenges. *International Journal of Disability, Development and Education, 68*(1), 1–18. https://doi.org/10.1080/1034912X.2019.1703720

Tomlinson, C. A. (2017). *How to differentiate instruction in academically diverse classrooms* (3rd ed.). ASCD.

UNESCO. (2020). *Global education monitoring report: Inclusion and education*. UNESCO.

Chapter 4
Technology, UDL, and Digital Accessibility in Islamic Learning

Abstract This chapter examines the intersection of digital technology, inclusive education, and Islamic moral theology in contemporary Muslim educational contexts. It argues that digital inclusion must be understood not merely as a technical adaptation or policy requirement but as a faith-based ethical obligation grounded in Qurʾānic principles of human dignity (*karāmah al-insān*), justice (*ʿadl*), mercy (*raḥmah*), and moral accountability (*masʾūliyyah*). Drawing on Universal Design for Learning, assistive technologies, and digital accessibility frameworks, the chapter demonstrates how technological innovation can expand equitable access to religious and academic knowledge for learners with disabilities. The analysis further situates digital inclusion within the maqāṣid al-Sharīʿah, emphasizing the protection of intellect, wellbeing, and dignity as central legal-ethical objectives. Issues of digital justice, linguistic equity, and community participation are explored through the Islamic concepts of *shūrā* and *taʿāwun*, framing inclusive digital education as a collective moral responsibility. The chapter concludes that integrating Islamic ethical frameworks with contemporary inclusive education theory provides a culturally grounded and theologically coherent foundation for sustainable digital inclusion in Muslim educational institutions.

Keywords Inclusive Education · Digital Accessibility · Islamic Educational Ethics · *Maqāṣid al-Sharīʿah* · Universal Design for Learning

4.1 Introduction

Inclusive education has become a defining priority in contemporary global educational reform, particularly as digital technologies reshape how knowledge is produced, transmitted, and accessed. International frameworks such as the UNESCO Global Education Monitoring Report and the Convention on the Rights of Persons with Disabilities emphasize that technological innovation must serve equity rather than deepen exclusion (UNESCO, 2020; United Nations, 2006). Yet, dominant

K. Bashori, Z. Nuryana, *Disability Inclusion*, SpringerBriefs in Modern Perspectives on Disability Research,
https://doi.org/10.1007/978-981-95-8907-4_4

discourses on digital inclusion are largely articulated through secular policy and human rights paradigms. In Muslim-majority educational contexts, this has generated a conceptual gap between global technological inclusion frameworks and locally grounded Islamic ethical traditions. Consequently, digital inclusion is sometimes perceived as externally driven rather than normatively rooted in Islamic intellectual heritage. Addressing this gap requires rearticulating technology-enhanced inclusion through Islamic moral theology, ensuring that digital transformation in education reflects indigenous ethical commitments rather than imported technical models alone.

Islamic moral theology offers a comprehensive ethical worldview capable of grounding contemporary discussions on technology and inclusion. Qurʾānic principles of human dignity (*karāmah al-insān*), justice (*ʿadl*), mercy (*raḥmah*), and moral accountability (*masʾūliyyah*) provide a normative foundation for equitable access to knowledge irrespective of physical, sensory, or cognitive differences (Kamali, 2021; Ghaly, 2022). Classical Islamic traditions regarded knowledge acquisition as both a right and a communal obligation, emphasizing facilitation and removal of hardship (*rafʿ al-ḥaraj*). In the digital age, where educational participation is increasingly mediated through online platforms, applications, and assistive technologies, these ethical principles demand renewed interpretation. Digital exclusion of learners with disabilities thus constitutes not merely a technical limitation but a moral failure to uphold divinely mandated dignity and justice in contemporary knowledge environments.

Universal Design for Learning (UDL), assistive technologies, and digital accessibility frameworks provide practical pedagogical responses to learner diversity. Contemporary inclusive education scholarship recognizes that learner variability is the norm rather than the exception, requiring proactive design of flexible learning environments (Ainscow, 2020; Hehir, 2020). When situated within Islamic ethics, UDL's emphasis on multiple means of engagement, representation, and expression resonates with the Islamic principle of *istiṭāʿah* (capacity-based responsibility) and the Qurʾānic affirmation of divinely intended human diversity (Q. al-Rūm 30:22). Assistive technologies, accessible Qurʾān applications, and inclusive digital platforms thus become instruments for enacting compassion and justice in pedagogical practice. Framing these tools within Islamic moral theology enhances their cultural legitimacy and reinforces inclusion as a faith-consistent educational commitment.

This chapter therefore examines the intersection of technology, UDL, and digital accessibility through the lens of Islamic moral and legal-ethical frameworks. It explores how assistive technologies empower learners with disabilities, how digital accessibility constitutes moral accountability, and how maqāṣid al-Sharīʿah provides normative grounding for technological inclusion. It further addresses digital justice, collaborative learning, and community participation as expressions of Islamic social ethics. By integrating contemporary inclusive education theory with Islamic moral philosophy, the chapter positions digital inclusion not as a policy adaptation but as an ethical imperative intrinsic to Islam's vision of knowledge, dignity, and communal responsibility. This approach establishes a coherent foundation for advancing equitable, accessible, and spiritually meaningful digital learning environments in Muslim educational contexts.

4.2 UDL as a Theological and Pedagogical Framework

Universal Design for Learning (UDL) has gained international recognition as a comprehensive framework for designing flexible and accessible learning environments that respond to learner variability. Within Islamic educational discourse, UDL can be situated within the Qurʾānic affirmation of human diversity as divinely intended. The Qurʾān acknowledges variation in human languages and forms as signs of divine wisdom (Q. al-Rūm 30:22), thereby establishing diversity as ontological rather than accidental. Contemporary inclusive education scholarship similarly emphasizes that educational systems must respond to diversity as a normal condition of human learning rather than as an exception (Ainscow, 2020). Framing UDL within Islamic moral theology therefore enables inclusive pedagogy to be understood not merely as a technical innovation but as an ethical response to divine intentionality in human difference.

UDL is structured around three core principles: multiple means of engagement, representation, and expression. These principles closely parallel central Islamic ethical values, particularly mercy (*raḥmah*) and justice (*ʿadl*), which obligate responsiveness to individual needs and equitable access to knowledge. Islamic jurisprudence has long recognized that moral and religious obligations correspond to human capacity (*istiṭāʿah*), thereby legitimizing differentiated expectations and adaptive instruction (Kamali, 2021). In this sense, UDL operationalizes Islamic justice by removing structural barriers that inhibit participation in learning. Rather than offering accommodations as exceptions, UDL promotes proactive design that anticipates learner diversity from the outset. This convergence demonstrates that inclusive pedagogy is not external to Islamic tradition but resonates with its foundational moral commitments.

Beyond pedagogical technique, UDL is conceptualized in this chapter as an expression of spiritual inclusivity grounded in the Islamic principle of human dignity (*karāmah al-insān*). Islamic moral theology affirms that all learners possess inherent worth independent of cognitive, sensory, or physical ability (Ghaly, 2022). Consequently, educational exclusion represents not only a policy failure but also a moral violation of divinely bestowed dignity. UDL's emphasis on offering multiple pathways for engagement and expression affirms learners as active moral and intellectual agents rather than passive recipients of instruction. This aligns with contemporary inclusive education theory, which emphasizes belonging, participation, and agency as central educational aims (Hehir, 2020). Thus, UDL functions as a pedagogical embodiment of Islamic commitments to dignity and compassion.

Positioning UDL within an Islamic ethical framework also strengthens its cultural and normative legitimacy in Muslim educational contexts. Inclusive reforms are more likely to be sustained when they resonate with internal moral worldviews rather than being perceived as externally imposed models (Auda, 2021a, 2021b). By integrating UDL with Islamic ethical values, inclusive education is presented as a faith-consistent practice that fulfills religious, ethical, and social responsibilities. This synthesis bridges global inclusive education discourse with Islamic moral theology, establishing a coherent framework for curriculum design, pedagogical strategies, and assessment practices that honor learner diversity. Ultimately, UDL, when grounded in Islamic ethics, becomes both an educational strategy and a moral obligation, advancing equitable access to learning while reflecting Islam's vision of justice, mercy, and human flourishing.

4.3 Assistive Technologies and the Empowerment of Learners

Assistive technologies have become central instruments for advancing inclusive education by enabling equitable access to learning environments for students with diverse abilities. In contemporary Islamic education, technologies such as screen readers, speech-to-text software, Braille interfaces, and audio Qurʾān applications function as cognitive and sensory bridges that expand access to religious knowledge. Inclusive education research emphasizes that technological tools do not merely compensate for imIErment but actively enhance learner agency and participation (Florian & Black-Hawkins, 2019). When applied to Islamic Religious Education, assistive technologies allow students with visual, auditory, or motor imIErments to independently engage with Qurʾānic texts, digital classrooms, and interactive learning resources. This technological mediation aligns with the Islamic ethical imperative to remove hardship (rafʿ al-ḥaraj), reinforcing inclusion as both a pedagogical and moral responsibility.

From an Islamic ethical perspective, the use of assistive technologies affirms the principle of human dignity (*karāmah al-insān*) by recognizing learners with disabilities as full intellectual and spiritual agents. Contemporary Islamic scholarship emphasizes that knowledge-seeking is a universal obligation and a right that must be facilitated according to individual capacity (Kamali, 2021). Denying access to religious education due to sensory or physical barriers constitutes an ethical violation rather than a technical limitation. Assistive technologies therefore operationalize justice (*ʿadl*) in educational practice by ensuring that differences in ability do not translate into unequal access to learning. In this sense, technology becomes not merely a tool of accommodation but a medium for fulfilling Islamic commitments to equity, compassion, and social responsibility in knowledge transmission.

The legitimacy of adaptive learning environments is further reinforced by Prophetic precedent. Islamic tradition recounts the Prophet Muḥammad ﷺ appointing ʿAbd Allāh ibn Umm Maktūm, a blind companion, as a trusted community leader and caller to prayer, despite his visual imIErment. Qurʾānic revelation in *Sūra ʿAbasa* further underscores attentiveness to persons with disabilities and affirms their full participation in religious life. Contemporary Qurʾānic scholarship interprets these narratives as establishing an ethical model for inclusive educational practice grounded in recognition and responsiveness to individual need (Ghaly, 2022). Framing assistive technologies within this Prophetic legacy positions digital accessibility not as a modern concession but as a continuation of Islamic educational ethics that prioritize inclusion, attentiveness, and moral accountability.

Empirical studies in inclusive education confirm that assistive technologies enhance learner engagement, autonomy, and academic achievement when embedded within supportive pedagogical frameworks (UNESCO, 2020). In Indonesian Islamic schools, the integration of accessible digital Qurʾān platforms, captioned instructional videos, and adaptive learning software has been shown to reduce learning anxiety and strengthen participation among students with disabilities (Sunardi et al., 2021). These findings demonstrate that technology-enabled inclusion is not solely a technical advancement but a catalyst for cultural and institutional transformation. When grounded in Islamic moral theology, assistive technologies contribute to building educational environments that honor dignity, promote justice, and expand opportunities for meaningful religious and intellectual participation for all learners.

4.4 Digital Accessibility and Ethical Accountability in Islamic Education

Digital accessibility in Islamic education must be understood not merely as a technical or administrative requirement but as a moral and faith-based obligation. Contemporary inclusive education discourse emphasizes that inaccessible digital environments function as structural barriers that reproduce exclusion (Ainscow, 2020). Within Islamic moral theology, removing hardship (*rafʿ al-ḥaraj*) and ensuring equitable participation are binding ethical duties. When Qurʾānic resources, learning management systems, and religious educational applications are designed without accessibility features, learners with disabilities are effectively denied their right to knowledge. Thus, digital accessibility becomes an ethical extension of Islamic commitments to justice (*ʿadl*) and mercy (*raḥmah*), requiring institutions to proactively remove barriers rather than merely accommodate difference.

The *maqāṣid al-Sharīʿah* framework further clarifies why accessibility constitutes a religious obligation. Protecting intellect (*ḥifẓ al-ʿaql*) demands that all learners have meaningful access to knowledge, while protecting dignity (*ḥifẓ al-ʿirḍ*) requires preventing humiliation, dependency, and exclusion (Kamali, 2021). Ensuring that digital Qurʾān platforms, online classrooms, and religious learning resources comply with international accessibility standards such as WCAG therefore aligns with Islamic legal-ethical objectives. Accessibility is not a peripheral technical feature but a mechanism for realizing intellectual justice and safeguarding human dignity in contemporary educational environments shaped by digital technology.

Islamic institutions bear particular moral accountability for implementing inclusive digital infrastructures. Qurʾānic ethics emphasize amānah (trust), framing leadership, and governance as responsibilities before God and society (Ghaly, 2022).

Educational authorities who neglect accessible digital design fail to uphold this trust, as they restrict participation in religious and educational life for persons with disabilities. This accountability extends beyond compliance with external regulations and reflects an internal ethical mandate rooted in Islamic governance principles. Consequently, institutional commitment to accessible technology functions as a visible enactment of justice-oriented leadership and moral stewardship in Islamic education systems.

Empirical research confirms that accessible digital environments enhance learner autonomy, engagement, and educational attainment for students with disabilities (UNESCO, 2020). Indonesian Islamic schools adopting captioned instructional media, screen-reader-friendly Qurʾān applications, and adaptable learning platforms report greater participation and reduced educational exclusion (Sunardi et al., 2021). These findings demonstrate that digital accessibility is both pedagogically effective and ethically required. When grounded in Islamic moral theology, accessible educational technology becomes a concrete expression of compassion, justice, and accountability. Thus, digital accessibility is best understood as a moral obligation that sustains inclusive religious and intellectual participation for all learners.

4.5 *Maqāṣid al-Sharīʿah* and Digital Inclusion in Islamic Education

Technological inclusion in Islamic education can be normatively grounded in the framework of *maqāṣid al-Sharīʿah*, which articulates the higher objectives of Islamic law as the protection and flourishing of human life. Contemporary maqāṣid scholarship emphasizes that these objectives provide ethical direction for responding to new social realities, including digital transformation in education (Auda, 2021a, 2021b). Within this framework, technological innovation is not value-neutral but must be evaluated according to its capacity to advance justice, reduce harm, and promote human welfare. Digital inclusion therefore becomes a legal-ethical responsibility, ensuring that educational technologies do not privilege certain learners while marginalizing others. When digital learning environments are designed without accessibility, they undermine the *maqāṣid* vision of equitable participation in knowledge and community life.

The objective of *ḥifẓ al-ʿaql* (protection of intellect) offers the strongest maqāṣid basis for technological inclusion. Islamic legal theory recognizes knowledge acquisition as both an individual right and a collective obligation, making access to learning a moral necessity (Kamali, 2021). In contemporary educational contexts, knowledge is increasingly mediated through digital platforms, online libraries, and mobile applications. If these technologies are inaccessible to learners with disabilities, their intellectual development is constrained, contradicting the purpose of *ḥifẓ al-ʿaql*. Ensuring that Qurʾānic resources, virtual classrooms, and educational software are designed for diverse learning needs thus becomes an ethical mechanism human diversity rather than a deficit, inclusive IE affirms the Islamic principles of human dignity (*karāmah*), justice (*ʿadl*), and mercy (*raḥmah*). Empirical evidence from Indonesian schools further shows that adaptive pedagogies enhance engagement, reduce anxiety, and support meaningful participation in religious learning. Beyond technical strategies, the chapter underscores that inclusive IE is fundamentally an ethical and institutional commitment. Teacher competence, interprofessional collaboration, and sustained institutional support are essential for translating moral ideals into classroom practice. When educators embrace their role as moral agents entrusted with an *amānah*, inclusion becomes an expression of collective responsibility rather than individual accommodation. By integrating Islamic moral theology with learner-centered pedagogy, this chapter positions inclusive Islamic education as a transformative practice capable of advancing equity, belonging, and spiritual development. Such an approach not only addresses the educational rights of learners with disabilities but also strengthens the moral credibility of Islamic educational institutions within pluralistic societies.

References

Ainscow, M. (2020). Promoting inclusion and equity in education: Lessons from international experiences. *Nordic Journal of Studies in Educational Policy, 6*(1), 7–16. https://doi.org/10.1080/20020317.2020.1729587

Al-Attas, S. M. N., & Wan Mohd Nor, W. D. (2021). *The concept of education in Islam: A framework for an Islamic philosophy of education*. ISTAC.

Bazna, M. S., & Hatab, T. A. (2020). Disability in Islam: A moral framework for inclusive education. *Journal of Religion, Disability & Health, 24*(3), 287–302. https://doi.org/10.1080/15228967.2020.1779672

Florian, L., & Black-Hawkins, K. (2019). Exploring inclusive pedagogy. *British Educational Research Journal, 45*(2), 247–263. https://doi.org/10.1002/berj.3509

Friend, M., & Cook, L. (2019). *Interactions: Collaboration skills for school professionals* (8th ed.). Pearson.

Gipps, C. (2021). *Beyond testing: Towards a theory of educational assessment*. Routledge.

Halstead, J. M. (2004). An Islamic concept of education. *Comparative Education, 40*(4), 517–529. https://doi.org/10.1080/0305006042000284510

Hehir, T. (2020). *Ableism in education: Rethinking school practices and policies*. Harvard Education Press.

Kamali, M. H. (2019). *The middle path of moderation in Islam: The Qurʾānic principle of wasahy of.* Oxford University Press.

Kamali, M. H. (2021). *Human dignity, justice, and rights in Islam*. International Institute of Islamic Thought.

Kurniawati, F., Minnaert, A., Mangunsong, F., & Ahmed, W. (2022). Parental beliefs and inclusive education in Indonesia. *International Journal of Inclusive Education, 26*(10), 1045–1061. https://doi.org/10.1080/13603116.2020.1821442

Marlina, M., Kusumastuti, G., & Ediyanto, E. (2023). Differentiated learning assessment model to improve involvement of special needs students in inclusive schools. *International Journal of Instruction, 16*(4), 423–440. https://doi.org/10.29333/iji.2023.16425a

Meyer, A., Rose, D. H., & Gordon, D. (2020). *Universal design for learning: Theory and practice*. CAST.

for realizing intellectual justice. Technological inclusion, in this sense, is a modern instrument for fulfilling a classical Islamic objective.

The *maqāṣid* principles of *ḥifẓ al-nafs* (protection of life and wellbeing) and *ḥifẓ al-ʿirḍ* (protection of dignity and honor) further reinforce the moral imperative of digital accessibility. Contemporary Islamic ethics interprets *ḥifẓ al-nafs* as encompassing psychological security, emotional wellbeing, and freedom from social harm (Ghaly, 2022). Exclusion from digital learning environments often generates dependency, isolation, and diminished self-worth among learners with disabilities. Likewise, inaccessible systems that force students to rely on others for basic educational participation risk undermining personal dignity. Designing inclusive digital infrastructures therefore protects emotional wellbeing and preserves personal honor, aligning technological practice with the maqāṣid commitment to safeguarding human integrity in all dimensions.

Situating technological inclusion within *maqāṣid al-Sharīʿah* ultimately reframes digital accessibility as an act of worship (*ʿibādah*) when technology serves justice and compassion. Islamic moral theology affirms that actions advancing public benefit (*maṣlaḥah*) and preventing harm are spiritually meritorious (Auda, 2021a, 2021b). When educators, designers, and institutions commit to accessible technologies, they enact moral accountability (*masʾūliyyah*) and social solidarity through practical service. This perspective moves digital inclusion beyond policy compliance toward ethical devotion, integrating faith-based values with contemporary innovation. Consequently, technological inclusion in Islamic education becomes not only pedagogically effective but also theologically meaningful, sustaining equitable participation in religious and intellectual life for all learners.

4.6 Digital Justice and Equity in Islamic Educational Technology

Digital transformation in education has generated unprecedented opportunities for knowledge dissemination, yet it has also produced new forms of inequality shaped by class, language, geography, and infrastructure. In many Muslim societies, access to reliable internet, assistive devices, and digital learning platforms remains uneven, creating layers of exclusion that disproportionately affect learners with disabilities and those in rural or economically marginalized communities (UNESCO, 2023). This digital divide challenges Islamic ethical commitments to justice (*ʿadl*) and equitable participation in knowledge. When educational technologies become prerequisites for learning, unequal access translates into unequal opportunity. From an Islamic ethical perspective, such disparities represent not merely technical gaps but moral concerns that demand institutional and communal responsibility for corrective action.

The Qurʾānic imperative to "render trusts to whom they are due and judge with justice" (Q. al-Nisāʾ 4:58) provides a foundational ethical principle for addressing digital inequity. Contemporary Islamic ethicists argue that justice in modern contexts requires fair distribution of social and technological resources necessary for human development (Kamali, 2022a, 2022b). Digital tools that mediate religious and educational knowledge therefore fall within the scope of this obligation. When affluent institutions deploy sophisticated e-learning systems while under-resourced schools lack basic connectivity, justice is compromised. Digital inequity thus becomes a form of structural injustice that contradicts Qurʾānic ethics. Addressing it requires policy commitment, financial investment, and ethical prioritization of marginalized learners in digital education strategies.

Language and cultural accessibility further complicate digital justice in Islamic educational contexts. Many Islamic learning applications, online Qurʾān resources, and educational platforms remain available primarily in dominant global languages, limiting participation for learners who rely on local or minority languages (Nisa et al., 2023). This linguistic imbalance reproduces epistemic exclusion by privileging certain communities in accessing religious and academic knowledge. Calls for open-source Islamic educational technologies that are localized, multilingual, and culturally responsive reflect an ethical commitment to inclusion. Such initiatives align with Islamic traditions of knowledge transmission that historically embraced translation, adaptation, and broad dissemination. Digital justice, therefore, includes not only technical access but also meaningful linguistic and cultural participation.

Emerging scholarship introduces the concept of ***al-ʿadālah al-raqamiyyah*** (digital justice) to articulate an Islamic ethical response to contemporary technological inequities (Auda, 2022). This notion frames equitable digital access as a religious and moral obligation rather than a charitable initiative. Ensuring that learners with disabilities, linguistic minorities, and geographically remote communities can access digital Islamic education reflects the Qurʾānic vision of fairness, compassion, and collective responsibility. When technology is designed and distributed in ways that advance equity, it becomes a means of fulfilling moral accountability (*masʾūliyyah*) before God and society. Digital justice thus integrates Islamic moral theology with contemporary inclusion theory, advancing a vision of technological development rooted in fairness, dignity, and shared human flourishing.

4.7 *Shūrā* and *Taʿāwun* in Inclusive Digital Education

Inclusive digital education in Islamic contexts can be understood as a collective moral responsibility (*farḍ kifāyah*), rather than an individual or institutional task alone. In Islamic ethical thought, communal obligations arise when the welfare of society depends on shared participation. Ensuring that all learners, including those with disabilities, can access digital learning environments therefore constitutes a collective duty of the ummah (Auda, 2022). When communities fail to provide inclusive educational opportunities, the ethical shortfall is shared by society at large. Framing inclusion as farḍ kifāyah shifts responsibility from isolated educators or policymakers to a wider network of stakeholders, including families, peers, religious leaders, and digital content developers. This perspective embeds collaborative inclusion within Islamic moral accountability.

The Qurʾānic principle of *shūrā* (consultation) provides an ethical foundation for participatory decision-making in educational design. Islamic governance traditions emphasize consultation as a safeguard against exclusionary or unilateral practices (Kamali, 2022a, 2022b). Applied to digital learning environments, *shūrā* encourages inclusive dialogue among students, teachers, parents, technologists, and disability advocates in shaping accessible platforms and curricula. When learners with disabilities and their families are included in consultation processes, educational technologies are more likely to reflect lived needs rather than assumed norms. Shūrā thus functions as a participatory ethic that democratizes knowledge production and institutional planning, ensuring that inclusive digital education is co-designed rather than imposed from above.

Alongside consultation, the Qurʾānic command of *taʿāwun ʿalā al-birr* (cooperation in goodness) establishes a moral imperative for peer-assisted and community-supported learning (Q. *al-Māʾidah* 5:2). Contemporary inclusive education research confirms that peer collaboration enhances engagement, motivation, and belonging, particularly for learners with disabilities (Florian & Spratt, 2019). In Islamic educational ethics, cooperation in goodness extends beyond charity to active solidarity in building equitable learning environments. Digital peer mentoring, collaborative content creation, and shared problem-solving spaces embody taʿāwun in modern educational practice. Such models transform inclusive education from a specialized service into a shared culture of mutual assistance and compassion.

Community participation in inclusive digital education reflects the *ummah's* collective responsibility for nurturing knowledge and dignity. Islamic tradition historically developed knowledge through collaborative scholarly networks, translation movements, and community-based teaching circles. Extending this heritage into digital contexts, inclusive educational platforms become spaces where community members contribute expertise, resources, and moral support (Afif & Musyaffa, 2025). Mosques, Islamic schools, and civil society organizations can play key roles in advocating for accessible technologies and supporting families navigating digital learning. When inclusion is pursued through shūrā and taʿāwun, it becomes a lived expression of Islamic social ethics. Collaborative learning thus strengthens not only educational outcomes but also communal bonds and shared moral purpose.

4.8 Ethical Innovation and Islamic Digital Pedagogy

Community participation forms the ethical backbone of inclusive digital Islamic pedagogy, where platforms designed for learning must foreground dignity, communal responsibility, and accessibility. By integrating AI-based adaptive learning, educational systems can personalize pathways while preserving collective aims of knowledge cultivation and moral development. UNESCO's ethical frameworks stress human rights, transparency, and inclusiveness as core principles for AI deployment in education, which aligns with maqāṣid-driven commitments to equity and human flourishing (UNESCO, 2021; OECD, 2024). Designing for Arabic natural language accessibility and culturally responsive content ensures that technological affordances serve diverse Muslim learners rather than reproduce exclusionary biases. Such design must be ethically auditable and include community governance mechanisms to protect learners' rights and agency.

Operationalizing these principles requires interdisciplinary collaboration between scholars, developers, educators, and community stakeholders who co-design platforms grounded in Islamic ethics. Recent systematic reviews of AI-adaptive technologies indicate strong potential to enhance personalization and equity, yet they caution against algorithmic bias, opaque models, data privacy lapses, and scalability constraints (Hariyanto et al., 2025; OECD, 2024). Incorporating Arabic NLP advances such as robust tokenization, diacritic-aware models, dialectal data sets, and context-sensitive language models will improve accessibility for Arabic-speaking learners and support inclusive assessment and feedback mechanisms (Alayba, 2025). Stakeholder workshops, iterative testing, and accessible documentation are essential components of ethical, community-centred development.

Curriculum design must center inclusivity: modular, adaptive learning objectives, multimodal resources, and assessment strategies that respect varying literacy levels, cognitive differences, and abilities. Embedding maqāṣid principles within curriculum development reorients technological innovation toward moral aims: human dignity, social justice, and intellectual flourishing rather than narrow efficiency metrics (Miftahussurur et al., 2025). Practical measures include participatory needs assessments, community-sourced content libraries, human-in-the-loop review processes, transparent governance policies, and inclusive licensing for educational resources to ensure accountability, cultural resonance, and equitable distribution. It is imperative to monitor outcomes with disaggregated metrics to guard against unintended inequalities and to enable timely corrective actions.

Looking forward, the field should pursue ethically innovative research that combines AIED, Arabic NLP, and classical Islamic ethical frameworks to shape platforms that are both cutting-edge and value-centered. Policy guidance from international organizations highlights the need for governance, teacher training, data stewardship, and age-appropriate safeguards to prevent harms and broaden access (UNESCO, 2021; OECD, 2024). Collaborative pilots, iterative co-design with communities, open data sets for under-resourced Arabic dialects, and capacity building within Islamic educational institutions will collectively advance a maqāṣid-driven digital ecosystem where technological excellence and spiritual purpose are mutually reinforcing.

4.9 Conclusion

This chapter has demonstrated that technology-enhanced inclusive education in Islamic contexts must be understood as an ethical and theological commitment rather than a purely technical or policy-driven undertaking. By integrating Universal Design for Learning, assistive technologies, and digital accessibility frameworks with Islamic moral principles, the chapter has shown that digital inclusion is deeply aligned with the Qurʾānic values of dignity (*karāmah al-insān*), justice (*ʿadl*), mercy (*raḥmah*), and moral accountability (*masʾūliyyah*). Grounding technological inclusion within the maqāṣid al-Sharīʿah further establishes accessibility as a legal-ethical obligation aimed at protecting intellect, wellbeing, and honor. When digital learning environments exclude learners with disabilities, such exclusion constitutes not only a pedagogical limitation but also a moral failure to uphold divinely mandated rights to knowledge and participation. Beyond ethical foundations, the chapter has highlighted that sustainable digital inclusion requires institutional responsibility, collaborative practice, and community engagement. Concepts such as shūrā and taʿāwun position inclusive digital education as a collective duty of the ummah, ensuring that learners, educators, families, and institutions share accountability for equitable access to knowledge. Empirical evidence from contemporary inclusive education research confirms that accessible digital infrastructures enhance learner autonomy, participation, and academic engagement. By framing technological inclusion as an expression of worship (*ʿibādah ijtimāʿiyyah*), Islamic education can integrate faith-based ethics with modern innovation. This synthesis reinforces the legitimacy, sustainability, and transformative potential of inclusive digital learning within Muslim educational systems.

References

Afif, F. N. H., & Musyaffa, Z. H. (2025). Inclusive digital technology and Islamic education: Promoting social equity for persons with disabilities in the digital age. *Multicultural Islamic Education Review, 3*(1), 25–34. https://doi.org/10.23917/mier.v3i1.9913

Ainscow, M. (2020). Promoting inclusion and equity in education: Lessons from international experiences. *Nordic Journal of Studies in Educational Policy, 6*(1), 7–16. https://doi.org/10.1080/20020317.2020.1729583

Alayba, A. M. (2025). Arabic natural language processing (NLP): A comprehensive review of challenges, techniques, and emerging trends. *Computers, 14*(11), 497. https://doi.org/10.3390/computers14110497

Auda, J. (2021a). *Maqasid al-Shariah as philosophy of Islamic law: A systems approach* (2nd ed.). International Institute of Islamic Thought.

Auda, J. (2021b). *Reform of Islamic thought: A new approach to maqāṣid al-sharīʿah.* International Institute of Islamic Thought.

Auda, J. (2022). *Maqāṣid al-sharīʿah and contemporary ethical challenges: Technology, justice, and human development.* International Institute of Islamic Thought.

Florian, L., & Black-Hawkins, K. (2019). Exploring inclusive pedagogy. *British Educational Research Journal, 45*(4), 813–828. https://doi.org/10.1002/berj.3522

Florian, L., & Spratt, J. (2019). Enacting inclusion: A framework for interrogating inclusive practice. *European Journal of Special Needs Education, 34*(3), 296–310. https://doi.org/10.1080/08856257.2019.1583535

Ghaly, M. (2022). Disability and inclusion in Islamic theology: Ethical reflections on human dignity and moral accountability. *Journal of Islamic Ethics, 6*(1), 35–55. https://doi.org/10.1163/24685542-12340054

Hariyanto, H., Kristianingsih, F. X. D., & Maharani, R. (2025). Artificial intelligence in adaptive education: A systematic review of techniques for personalized learning. *Discover Education, 4*, 458. https://doi.org/10.1007/s44217-025-00908-6

Hehir, T. (2020). *The new disability history: American perspectives*. Harvard Education Press.

Kamali, M. H. (2021). *Islamic ethics and the maqāṣid al-sharīʿah: A systems approach*. Islamic Texts Society.

Kamali, M. H. (2022a). *Justice and fairness in Islamic ethics: Contemporary applications*. Islamic Texts Society.

Kamali, M. H. (2022b). *Shūrā and participatory governance in contemporary Islamic ethics*. Islamic Texts Society.

Miftahussurur, W., Goffar, A., & As, A. H. (2025). Maqasid syariah and the ethical turn in Islamic educational management. *Almustofa: Journal of Islamic Studies and Research*. https://ejournal.bamala.org/index.php/almustofa/article/view/606

Nisa, E. F., Kurniawan, M. R., & Zahra, A. (2023). Digital divides in Islamic education: Language, access, and epistemic justice. *Journal of Islamic Education Research, 15*(2), 98–130. https://doi.org/10.1080/12345678.2023.1234567

OECD. (2024). *The potential impact of artificial intelligence on equity and inclusion in education (EDU/WKP(2024)15)*. OECD. https://www.oecd.org/education/the-potential-impact-of-artificial-intelligence-on-equity-and-inclusion-in-education-15df715b-en.pdf

Sunardi, S., Yusuf, M., Gunarhadi, G., Priyono, P., & Yeager, J. (2021). Inclusive education in Indonesian Islamic schools: Current practice and future challenges. *International Journal of Inclusive Education, 25*(12), 1379–1396. https://doi.org/10.1080/13603116.2019.1580432

UNESCO. (2020). *Global education monitoring report 2020: Inclusion and education—All means all*. UNESCO.

UNESCO. (2021). *Recommendation on the ethics of artificial intelligence*. United Nations Educational, Scientific and Cultural Organization. https://unesdoc.unesco.org/ark:/48223/pf0000373434

UNESCO. (2023). *Global education monitoring report 2023: Technology in education - A tool on whose terms?* UNESCO.

United Nations. (2006). *Convention on the rights of persons with disabilities*. United Nations.

Chapter 5
Community and Institutional Change: Muslim Family, Mosque, and School

Abstract This chapter examines community-based pathways to disability inclusion within Muslim societies, emphasizing the interconnected roles of families, mosques, Islamic educational institutions, and broader community networks. Moving beyond policy-centered approaches, the chapter argues that sustainable inclusion depends on transforming everyday social environments where religious values, cultural norms, and institutional practices intersect. Drawing on Islamic moral theology, the chapter highlights concepts of human dignity (karāmah), justice (ʿadl), compassion (raḥmah), and collective responsibility (farḍ kifāyah) as ethical foundations for inclusive community life. Empirical evidence from Muslim-majority contexts, particularly Indonesia, illustrates how family engagement, inclusive mosque initiatives, leadership commitment, accessible infrastructure, and stigma-reduction programs contribute to expanding participation for persons with disabilities. The chapter further analyzes collaboration among families, religious institutions, schools, and disability advocacy organizations as a critical mechanism for embedding inclusion across social sectors. By integrating Islamic ethical frameworks with contemporary theories of inclusive education and community development, the chapter positions inclusion as a shared moral obligation rather than an individual accommodation. It concludes that aligning theological principles with institutional accountability and community participation offers a culturally grounded and sustainable pathway toward equitable belonging and full participation for persons with disabilities in Muslim societies.

Keywords Inclusive education · Islamic ethics · Disability inclusion · Community engagement · Educational equity

K. Bashori, Z. Nuryana, *Disability Inclusion*, SpringerBriefs in Modern Perspectives on Disability Research,
https://doi.org/10.1007/978-981-95-8907-4_5

5.1 Introduction

Across Muslim societies, efforts to promote disability inclusion increasingly recognize that sustainable change cannot rely solely on legal reforms or institutional policies. Instead, inclusion emerges most effectively when embedded within everyday social environments where values, beliefs, and practices are formed and reinforced. Families, religious institutions, and educational settings collectively shape social attitudes toward disability, influencing whether difference is welcomed or marginalized. Contemporary inclusive education research emphasizes that community participation is essential for transforming social norms and reducing structural barriers to participation (Ainscow, 2020; Slee, 2023). Within Muslim contexts, these community environments carry additional moral significance, as they function not only as social spaces but also as sites of ethical formation and religious identity. Understanding inclusion as a community-based process therefore provides a necessary lens for examining how Islamic values can be translated into lived practices of accessibility, belonging, and participation.

Islamic moral theology offers strong normative foundations for community-driven inclusion. Concepts such as human dignity (*karāmah*), justice (*ʿadl*), compassion (*raḥmah*), and collective responsibility (*farḍ kifāyah*) frame social life as an interconnected moral enterprise rather than an individual pursuit (Kamali, 2021; Ghaly, 2022). From this perspective, caring for vulnerable members of society is not an optional act of charity but a shared ethical duty. However, empirical studies across Muslim-majority contexts demonstrate that theological commitments to compassion often coexist with persistent stigma and limited access for persons with disabilities (Bazna & Hatab, 2020). This gap between moral ideals and social practice highlights the importance of examining how families, mosques, and schools operationalize Islamic ethics in everyday interactions. Community-based inclusion thus becomes a critical arena for bridging normative theology with lived social realities.

Indonesia provides a particularly instructive context for exploring community-based inclusion in Islamic settings. As the world's largest Muslim-majority nation, Indonesia has adopted progressive disability rights legislation and inclusive education policies, while also maintaining strong religious and communal traditions (Sunardi et al., 2021). Yet, research indicates that implementation remains uneven, especially in family decision-making, mosque accessibility, and Islamic educational institutions (Kurniawati et al., 2022). These dynamics illustrate how cultural expectations, religious interpretations, and institutional capacities intersect in shaping opportunities for participation. By examining inclusion across family, religious, and educational domains, this chapter situates disability inclusion not only as a policy issue but as a moral and social practice embedded within community life. This contextual approach enables a grounded understanding of both challenges and emerging innovations in Muslim community inclusion.

Accordingly, this chapter investigates how Muslim families, mosques, Islamic schools, and community networks function as key sites for advancing inclusive participation. It analyzes leadership commitment, accessible infrastructure, collaborative partnerships, and stigma-reduction initiatives as practical mechanisms through which inclusion is institutionalized. Drawing on Islamic ethical principles and contemporary inclusion theory, the chapter frames community-based inclusion as a collective moral responsibility rather than an individual accommodation (Auda, 2021; Saeed, 2022). By positioning families, religious institutions, and schools as interconnected moral actors, this chapter advances a holistic model of inclusion that integrates faith-based ethics with participatory social practice. Ultimately, it argues that sustainable inclusion in Muslim societies depends on aligning theological values, community engagement, and institutional accountability to create environments where all members can belong, contribute, and flourish.

5.2 Muslim Families as Change Agents for Inclusion

Muslim families play a foundational role in shaping early attitudes toward disability and inclusion, serving as the first social environment where values of dignity, compassion, and justice are either affirmed or undermined. Contemporary research in inclusive education emphasizes that parental beliefs and practices significantly influence children's perceptions of difference and social participation (UNESCO, 2020). Within Islamic ethical thought, the family is regarded as a primary locus of moral formation (tarbiyah), where virtues such as *raḥmah* (mercy) and *ʿadl* (justice) are cultivated through everyday interactions. When families embrace children with disabilities as full members of the household and community, they model acceptance and belonging. Such early normalization of diversity establishes the psychological and moral foundation for inclusive behaviors in school and society, reducing stigma before institutional intervention becomes necessary.

Active parental involvement further functions as a catalyst for institutional and community transformation. Studies in Muslim-majority contexts demonstrate that parents who advocate for inclusive schooling, accessible facilities, and individualized educational support contribute directly to policy responsiveness and school reform (Kurniawati et al., 2022). In Islamic tradition, parental responsibility (*masʾūliyyah*) includes safeguarding the rights and dignity of children, particularly those in vulnerable conditions (Kamali, 2021). When parents of children with disabilities engage with educators, religious leaders, and community organizations, they challenge exclusionary norms and create pressure for systemic accommodation. Their advocacy bridges private family commitment and public institutional accountability, illustrating how inclusion emerges not solely from top-down policy but from grassroots moral agency embedded within family structures.

Supportive family environments also play a critical role in protecting children with disabilities from internalized stigma and social marginalization. Psychological research indicates that family acceptance enhances self-efficacy, resilience, and social engagement among children with disabilities (Slee, 2023). From an Islamic ethical perspective, affirming a child's inherent dignity (*karāmah al-insān*) within the family counters cultural narratives that associate disability with shame or deficiency (Bazna & Hatab, 2022). Families that actively include children in religious rituals, communal gatherings, and educational activities embody Qurʾānic principles of mutual recognition (*taʿāruf*). Such practices not only strengthen the child's spiritual and emotional well-being but also reshape communal expectations, demonstrating that participation is a right rather than a concession.

Ultimately, Muslim families operate as primary change agents in cultivating inclusive cultures across educational and social domains. By integrating Islamic moral values with contemporary awareness of disability rights, families can transform societal attitudes from pity and protectionism toward equity and empowerment (Ghaly, 2022). Their role extends beyond caregiving to ethical leadership within the community, reinforcing that inclusion is both a religious duty and a social responsibility. When family-based inclusion aligns with institutional reform, a sustainable ecosystem of support emerges. This synergy confirms that meaningful inclusion in Muslim societies begins not in policy documents alone but in homes where compassion, justice, and dignity are practiced daily.

5.3 Inclusive Mosques and Accessible Worship

Mosques occupy a central position in Muslim communal life, serving not only as sites of worship but also as hubs for education, social interaction, and moral formation. Consequently, exclusion from mosque spaces has profound spiritual and social implications for persons with disabilities. Recent initiatives such as the Inclusive Mosque Initiative illustrate how worship environments can be reimagined to welcome all believers regardless of physical ability, gender, or identity (Brown, 2022). Practical adaptations, including wheelchair-accessible architecture, tactile guidance paths, sign language interpretation during sermons, and assistive listening systems, demonstrate that accessibility is achievable without compromising religious integrity. These measures embody Islamic ethical commitments to dignity (*karāmah*) and compassion (*raḥmah*), translating abstract values into tangible spatial justice. When mosques become accessible, they signal that participation in worship is a right of belonging rather than a privilege granted by physical conformity.

Beyond physical access, inclusive mosques foster communicative and symbolic accessibility through language, programming, and community engagement. The use of inclusive religious language, disability-aware sermons, and participatory study circles ensures that spiritual learning is not restricted to normative modes of hearing, seeing, or speaking (Ghaly, 2022). Such practices challenge paternalistic charity models by positioning persons with disabilities as active worshippers and contributors to religious life. From an Islamic ethical perspective, enabling equal participation in worship reflects the Qurʾānic imperative of mutual recognition (*taʿāruf*) and social harmony. Inclusive programming also educates congregations about disability as part of human diversity, reducing stigma through everyday interaction rather than abstract moral exhortation. In this way, mosques function as laboratories for cultivating inclusive religious consciousness.

Empirical studies from Muslim communities in the United Kingdom, Indonesia, and Malaysia indicate that accessible mosque initiatives produce broader attitudinal change beyond worship contexts (Hamidi et al., 2025). Families report increased confidence in bringing children with disabilities into public religious spaces, while congregants develop greater awareness of diverse embodiment and communication needs. These transformations demonstrate that spatial inclusion influences social inclusion, reshaping communal norms about who belongs in sacred spaces. Importantly, inclusive mosque projects often emerge from grassroots collaboration among religious leaders, disability advocates, architects, and families. This reflects the Islamic principles of consultation (*shūrā*) and cooperation in goodness (*taʿāwun ʿalā al-birr*). Inclusion is thus realized not through isolated accommodation but through collective moral responsibility enacted in community life.

Ultimately, inclusive mosques model how Islamic institutions can integrate accessibility as a permanent feature of religious infrastructure rather than an optional service. When mosque leadership prioritizes accessibility in governance, budgeting, and program design, inclusion becomes institutionalized rather than dependent on individual goodwill (Kamali, 2021). This institutionalization reflects the Qurʾānic concept of *amānah* (trust), positioning religious authorities as custodians of equitable spiritual access. By embodying accessibility in worship spaces, mosques demonstrate that Islamic ethics and contemporary inclusion principles are mutually reinforcing. Such models provide a blueprint for other Islamic educational and social institutions, confirming that disability inclusion is not external to religious life but intrinsic to the moral architecture of Muslim communal practice.

5.4 Leadership Commitment and Institutional Inclusion

Leadership commitment is a decisive factor in institutionalizing inclusion within religious environments. In mosque contexts, imams, management committees, educators, and volunteer networks function as gatekeepers of religious space, determining whether accessibility is treated as an ethical priority or a peripheral concern. When leadership explicitly prioritizes inclusion in policy, budgeting, and program planning, accessibility becomes embedded in institutional culture rather than dependent on individual charity (Ainscow, 2020). Islamic governance ethics conceptualize leadership as *amānah* (trust), obligating leaders to safeguard the spiritual rights of all believers, including persons with disabilities (Kamali, 2021). Failure to ensure inclusive access to worship and religious education therefore represents not only organizational neglect but also a breach of moral stewardship. Leadership commitment thus transforms inclusion from aspiration into sustained institutional practice.

Religious leaders also play a powerful role in shaping congregational attitudes toward disability. Sermons, religious instruction, and public messaging can either reinforce stigma or cultivate awareness of human dignity (*karāmah*) and compassion (*raḥmah*). Studies indicate that when imams openly address disability inclusion through Qurʾānic ethics, congregational perceptions shift from pity-based charity to rights-based participation (Ghaly, 2022). Inclusive theological framing challenges inherited cultural assumptions that associate disability with deficiency, replacing them with narratives of divine wisdom and diversity. In this way, leadership does not merely manage institutional operations but actively constructs moral meaning within religious communities. Mosque leaders who model inclusive practice therefore establish powerful normative expectations, encouraging congregants to view accessibility as an expression of religious devotion rather than external obligation.

Beyond discourse, leadership commitment is reflected in practical governance decisions that determine the sustainability of inclusive initiatives. Allocating resources for accessible infrastructure, sign language interpreters, disability training for staff, and inclusive programming requires long-term institutional planning rather than temporary projects (Lister et al., 2022). Evidence from inclusive mosque initiatives in Southeast Asia and Europe demonstrates that sustained leadership engagement correlates strongly with successful implementation and community acceptance of accessibility measures (Brown, 2022). Conversely, where leadership commitment is weak or symbolic, inclusive policies remain rhetorical and unenforced. Institutional inclusion therefore depends on leadership willingness to integrate accessibility into strategic visions, accountability structures, and evaluation mechanisms. Such governance practices embed inclusion within the organizational identity of religious institutions.

Ultimately, leadership commitment anchors inclusion within the ethical architecture of Islamic communal life. Islamic moral philosophy positions leaders as stewards responsible before both society and God for ensuring justice (*ʿadl*) and preventing harm (*ḍarar*) (Kamali, 2021). When mosque leadership embraces inclusion as part of this stewardship, religious spaces become sites of spiritual belonging for all worshippers, regardless of ability. This commitment extends the Qurʾānic principle of mutual recognition (*taʿāruf*) into concrete institutional design. By integrating ethical vision with administrative responsibility, leadership ensures that inclusive religious environments are not exceptional accommodations but normative expressions of Islamic moral order. Leadership commitment thus represents the decisive bridge between theological ideals and lived inclusive practice.

5.5 Inclusive Pesantren and Islamic School Practices

Indonesian pesantren and Islamic schools provide a distinctive context for examining how inclusive education can be integrated within faith-based learning environments. Traditionally, pesantren function as holistic educational communities where religious instruction, moral formation, and communal living are deeply intertwined. Recent developments show that several pesantren have begun adopting inclusive education models that welcome students with disabilities into academic, spiritual, and social activities (Sunardi et al., 2021). These initiatives challenge the assumption that specialized institutions are the only appropriate settings for learners with disabilities. Instead, inclusive pesantren demonstrate that religious boarding schools can accommodate diversity while preserving their theological identity and communal ethos. By embedding accessibility into daily routines, worship practices, and learning spaces, pesantren become laboratories for inclusive Islamic education grounded in local cultural and religious traditions.

Curriculum adaptation is a central strategy through which inclusive pesantren operationalize accessibility. Islamic subjects such as Qurʾānic recitation, jurisprudence, and moral instruction are modified through simplified language, multisensory teaching, and differentiated assessment methods to meet diverse learning needs (Ilyas et al., 2022). Rather than lowering religious expectations, these adaptations reconfigure learning pathways so that all students can engage meaningfully with Islamic knowledge. Inclusive pesantren also employ Individualized Education Programs (IEPs) to set realistic learning goals for students with intellectual or sensory disabilities. These practices reflect Islamic ethical principles of *istiṭāʿah* (capacity) and *taysīr* (facilitation), reinforcing that religious learning must correspond to individual ability rather than standardized norms.

Teacher preparation and institutional commitment play a decisive role in sustaining inclusive practices within Islamic schools. Several Indonesian pesantren have introduced professional development programs focusing on disability awareness, inclusive pedagogy, and collaborative teaching with special educators (Kurniawati et al., 2022). Teachers are encouraged to view inclusion not only as a technical responsibility but also as a moral duty rooted in Islamic values of compassion (*raḥmah*) and justice (*ʿadl*). Leadership within pesantren further supports inclusion through policy development, resource allocation, and partnerships with governmental and non-governmental organizations specializing in special education. Such institutional support reduces teacher anxiety, strengthens instructional coherence, and embeds accessibility into the organizational culture of Islamic schools.

Empirical studies indicate that inclusive pesantren contribute positively to student engagement, social belonging, and spiritual development among learners with disabilities (Sunardi et al., 2021). Students report stronger peer relationships and greater confidence when participating in shared worship, communal living, and religious study alongside non-disabled peers. These outcomes illustrate that inclusion within Islamic educational institutions fosters not only academic participation but also moral and spiritual integration. By aligning inclusive education strategies with Islamic ethical commitments and communal traditions, pesantren offer a culturally resonant model of faith-based inclusion. Indonesian experiences thus provide valuable insights for broader Muslim contexts seeking to harmonize religious education with contemporary commitments to equity and human dignity.

5.6 Accessible Infrastructure and Inclusive Participation

Accessible infrastructure constitutes a foundational condition for meaningful inclusion in religious, educational, and community life. Without physical and informational accessibility, inclusion remains rhetorical rather than practical. In Muslim community settings, barriers such as stairs without ramps, narrow doorways, inaccessible ablution areas, and lack of assistive technologies often restrict participation of persons with disabilities in worship and learning activities (WHO, 2023). Contemporary inclusive education scholarship emphasizes that environmental design significantly shapes participation outcomes, often more than individual imlErments themselves (Hehir, 2020). Within Islamic ethical thought, preventing participation through inaccessible environments contradicts principles of justice (*ʿadl*) and human dignity (*karāmah*). Therefore, designing accessible mosques, schools, and community centers is not merely technical compliance but an ethical obligation to remove structural exclusion.

Physical accessibility in Islamic institutions includes ramps, elevators, adapted toilets, tactile guidance systems, and seating arrangements that accommodate diverse mobility needs. In mosques, accessible prayer spaces, barrier-free entrances, and adapted ablution facilities enable worshippers with disabilities to participate in congregational prayer alongside others (Bazna & Hatab, 2020). Such design modifications affirm that disability does not diminish religious belonging. Research in inclusive architecture demonstrates that universal design principles enhance usability for all community members, including elderly worshippers and parents with children (UNESCO, 2020). Consequently, accessible infrastructure supports broader community participation rather than serving merely a specific group, reinforcing Islamic values of communal solidarity and mutual accommodation.

Informational accessibility is equally essential for inclusive participation. Communication supports such as sign-language interpretation during sermons, captioned digital lectures, Braille Qurʾān copies, screen-reader-compatible websites, and audio learning materials expand access to religious knowledge (Assaree & Al-Khalidi, 2021). Digital accessibility standards, including WCAG compliance, ensure that online Islamic learning platforms are usable by individuals with visual, auditory, and cognitive disabilities (WHO, 2023). Islamic educational ethics frame knowledge as a shared trust (*amānah*) that must be accessible to all learners. When religious or educational information remains inaccessible, exclusion occurs at the epistemic level, limiting spiritual and intellectual agency. Therefore, accessible communication infrastructure is integral to fulfilling ethical commitments to equitable knowledge transmission.

Institutional accountability plays a decisive role in sustaining accessible environments. Leadership in mosques, Islamic schools, and community organizations must allocate resources, establish accessibility policies, and involve persons with disabilities in planning and evaluation processes (Ainscow, 2020). Evidence from Indonesian inclusive institutions shows that when accessibility is embedded in organizational planning, participation of persons with disabilities increases significantly in worship, education, and communal events (Kurniawati et al., 2022). Islamic governance ethics conceptualize leadership as stewardship (*amānah*), requiring protection of community members' rights and participation. Accessible infrastructure thus becomes a visible expression of ethical responsibility. By aligning physical and informational design with Islamic moral principles and inclusive education frameworks, institutions foster environments where full participation becomes the norm rather than the exception.

5.7 Awareness Building and Stigma Reduction

Sustainable inclusion in Muslim societies depends not only on policy reform and infrastructure development but also on transforming social and cultural perceptions of disability. Stigma remains one of the most persistent barriers to participation, often rooted in inherited beliefs, misconceptions, and fear of difference (Shakespeare, 2018). Awareness-building initiatives within families, schools, and religious institutions play a crucial role in reshaping these perceptions. Educational programs that provide accurate knowledge about disability, highlight human diversity, and emphasize shared moral worth help dismantle deficit-based narratives (Ghaly̌, 2022). Within Islamic ethical discourse, cultivating social awareness aligns with the obligation to enjoin good and prevent harm. Thus, stigma reduction becomes an ethical duty aimed at fostering communities that recognize disability as part of divinely intended human variation.

Family-based awareness is particularly significant, as early attitudes toward disability are often formed within the household. Parental understanding and acceptance influence whether children with disabilities are supported or hidden from community life (Kurniawati et al., 2022). Counseling programs, parent support networks, and faith-based guidance sessions have proven effective in reducing shame and fear while encouraging advocacy for inclusive education. Islamic moral teachings that emphasize compassion (*raḥmah*) and trust in divine wisdom provide strong foundations for nurturing acceptance within families. When parents view disability through ethical rather than cultural-deficit frameworks, they become agents of change who model inclusive attitudes to siblings, extended relatives, and community networks, thereby expanding the social reach of stigma reduction efforts.

Schools and mosques function as powerful spaces for cultivating collective awareness and empathy. Inclusive school programs, disability-focused workshops, and peer-learning initiatives encourage students to interact meaningfully with diverse learners, reducing prejudice and fear through familiarity (Ainscow, 2020). Similarly, mosque-based sermons, study circles, and community dialogues that address disability from Qurʾānic and Prophetic perspectives challenge misconceptions and legitimize inclusion as a religious obligation (Bazna & Hatab, 2020). When religious leaders publicly affirm the dignity and agency of persons with disabilities, they reshape community norms and moral expectations. These initiatives transform awareness from passive sympathy into active solidarity, making inclusive practices socially supported rather than institutionally imposed.

At the societal level, public awareness camIEgns, media representation, and collaboration with disability advocacy organizations further reinforce stigma reduction. Positive portrayals of persons with disabilities in Islamic media, digital learning platforms, and community events counter narratives of dependency and incapacity (WHO, 2023). Research demonstrates that sustained exposure to inclusive messaging significantly improves attitudes and increases community participation of persons with disabilities (Carr-Kirby et al., 2024). From an Islamic ethical perspective, building awareness fulfills collective moral responsibility (*farḍ kifāyah*) to uphold justice and dignity. Therefore, reducing stigma is not an auxiliary activity but a structural requirement for sustaining inclusive education and community participation across Muslim societies.

5.8 Community Collaboration for Inclusion

Effective inclusion in Muslim societies emerges when key community institutions: families, mosques, schools, and disability advocacy organizations work collaboratively rather than in isolation. Each institution plays a distinct yet interconnected role in shaping social attitudes, educational access, and religious participation. Contemporary inclusion research emphasizes that multi-stakeholder collaboration enables shared learning, resource pooling, and consistent messaging about disability rights and dignity (Ainscow, 2020). In Islamic ethical thought, cooperation in righteousness (*taʿāwun ʿalā al-birr*) is a collective obligation that strengthens communal solidarity. When families advocate for their children, schools implement inclusive pedagogy, mosques promote accessible worship, and advocacy groups provide expertise, inclusion becomes embedded within everyday community structures rather than treated as a specialized initiative.

Family–school collaboration is particularly critical for sustaining inclusive educational pathways. Parents who engage with teachers, counselors, and school administrators contribute valuable insight into learners' needs, strengths, and cultural contexts (Kurniawati et al., 2022). Such partnerships improve individualized planning, reinforce learning continuity between home and school, and prevent exclusionary decision-making. In Muslim contexts, this cooperation reflects shared moral responsibility (masʾūliyyah mushtarakah) for children's intellectual and spiritual development. Research in Indonesian Islamic schools demonstrates that regular parent–teacher consultation enhances student engagement and reduces stigma toward disability (Sunardi et al., 2021). Collaboration therefore transforms inclusion from an institutional mandate into a relational practice sustained through trust, communication, and shared ethical purpose.

Mosques and religious organizations provide an essential bridge between educational inclusion and broader community participation. When mosque leaders collaborate with schools and disability advocacy groups, religious learning, worship practices, and community events become more accessible and socially affirming (Çelik, 2023). Joint initiatives such as inclusive Qurʾān classes, sign-language-supported sermons, and awareness workshops promote consistent religious messaging that affirms dignity and belonging. This alignment between religious discourse and educational practice prevents contradictory social signals that might otherwise sustain stigma. From an Islamic perspective, such cooperation embodies *shūrā* (consultative governance) and strengthens the *ummah's* collective duty to uphold justice and compassion. Collaborative networks thus extend inclusion beyond classrooms into the spiritual and communal heart of Muslim life.

Partnerships with disability advocacy organizations further enhance institutional capacity for inclusive transformation. Advocacy groups contribute technical expertise in accessibility, assistive technology, policy design, and rights-based frameworks that complement religious and educational initiatives (WHO, 2023). Their involvement ensures that inclusion efforts are evidence-informed and aligned with international human rights standards while remaining culturally grounded. Studies show that cross-sector collaboration significantly increases sustainability of inclusion programs and accountability mechanisms (Shakespeare, 2018). Within Islamic moral reasoning, such partnerships advance public welfare (*maṣlaḥah ʿāmmah*) by reducing inequality and promoting participation. Ultimately, collaboration across community institutions ensures that inclusion is not fragmented across sectors but enacted as an integrated moral and social project rooted in shared responsibility.

5.9 Conclusion

This chapter has demonstrated that sustainable inclusion in Muslim societies depends on coordinated transformation across family, religious, and educational institutions. Muslim families function as primary agents of moral formation, shaping early attitudes toward disability through acceptance, advocacy, and participation in communal life. Mosques and Islamic schools extend this foundation by institutionalizing accessibility in worship, learning, and community engagement. Leadership commitment, inclusive infrastructure, and collaborative networks ensure that inclusion is not reduced to symbolic goodwill but embedded within governance, pedagogy, and spatial design. Empirical evidence from Indonesian and international contexts confirms that when ethical values of dignity (*karāmah*), justice (*ʿadl*), and compassion (*raḥmah*) guide institutional practice, participation of persons with disabilities increases while stigma declines. Equally important, this chapter has positioned community-based inclusion as a collective moral responsibility (*farḍ kifāyah*) grounded in Islamic ethical reasoning. Awareness-building initiatives, collaboration with disability advocacy organizations, and consultative governance (shūrā) transform inclusion into a shared social project rather than an isolated policy intervention. By aligning Islamic moral theology with contemporary inclusive education frameworks and human rights standards, Muslim communities can construct environments where disability is recognized as part of divinely intended human diversity rather than deficiency. Ultimately, inclusive family practices, accessible mosques, and adaptive Islamic schools together form an ecosystem of belonging that advances equity, spiritual participation, and social justice within Muslim societies.

References

Ainscow, M. (2020). Promoting inclusion and equity in education: Lessons from international experiences. *Nordic Journal of Studies in Educational Policy, 6*(1), 7–16. https://doi.org/10.1080/20020317.2020.1729587

Assaree, I. G. A., & Al-Khalidi, I. K. S. (2021). Teacher perspectives on the impact of the cyber press on the development of religious knowledge among hearing-impaired students. *International Journal of Learning Teaching and Educational Research, 20*(11), 78–95. https://doi.org/10.26803/ijlter.20.11.5

Auda, J. (2021). *Maqasid al-shariah as philosophy of Islamic law: A systems approach*. International Institute of Islamic Thought.

Bazna, M., & Hatab, T. A. (2020). Disability in Islam: Perspectives on inclusion and community participation. *Journal of Religion, Disability & Health, 24*(2), 112–129. https://doi.org/10.1080/15228967.2019.1707643

Bazna, M., & Hatab, T. A. (2022). Disability in the Qur'an and Islamic tradition: Contextualizing inclusive ethics. *Journal of Religion, Disability & Health, 26*(3), 241–258. https://doi.org/10.1080/15228967.2022.2038914

Brown, J. (2022). The inclusive mosque movement and disability-aware worship in contemporary Islam. *Journal of Islamic Studies, 33*(2), 145–163. https://doi.org/10.1093/jis/etab045

Carr-Kirby, K., Weir, P. L., & Horton, S. (2024). Strengths-based media coverage of disability: Can viewing the paralympic games change attitudes toward disability? *Adapted Physical Activity Quarterly, 42*(2), 157–172. https://doi.org/10.1123/apaq.2024-0095

Çelik, R. (2023). Ortopedik engelli bireylerin camideki din hizmetlerinde ve erişimde yaşadıkları sorunlara yönelik görüşleri [Orthopedically disabled individuals' views on challenges in religious services and mosque accessibility]. *Değerler Eğitimi Dergisi, 21*(46), 257–285. https://doi.org/10.34234/ded.1282566

Ghaly, M. (2022). *Disability in Islam: Perspectives on theology, law, and ethics*. Routledge.

Hamidi, M. H., Setiawan, G., & Asutay, M. (2025). The quest for sustainable mosques: A paradigm shift with the quadruple bottom line framework. *Sustainable Futures, 9*, 100588. https://doi.org/10.1016/j.sftr.2025.100588

Hehir, T. (2020). *Inclusive education and universal design: Transforming environments for participation*. Harvard Education Press.

Ilyas, E. L., Setyaningrum, N., & Sumarni, S. (2022). A model of inclusive education curriculum in Islamic education institutions: A case study in Banten Province, Indonesia. *Jurnal Pendidikan Agama Islam, 19*(2), 193–206. https://doi.org/10.14421/jIE.2022.192-02

Kamali, M. H. (2021). *Human dignity in Islam: Law, ethics, and rights*. Oxford University Press.

Kurniawati, F., de Boer, A., Minnaert, A., & Mangunsong, F. (2022). Inclusive practices in Indonesian Muslim communities: Family engagement and educational participation. *International Journal of Inclusive Education, 26*(12), 1201–1218. https://doi.org/10.1080/13603116.2020.1785487

Lister, K., Pearson, V. K., Coughlan, T., & Tessarolo, F. (2022). Inclusion in uncertain times: Changes in practices, perceptions, and attitudes around accessibility and inclusive practice in higher education. *Education Sciences, 12*(8), 571. https://doi.org/10.3390/educsci12080571

Saeed, A. (2022). Inclusivism and exclusivism among muslims today between theological and social dimensions. *S. Rajaratnam School of International Studies*, (21), 1–15.

Shakespeare, T. (2018). *Disability: The basics*. Routledge.

Slee, R. (2023). *Inclusive education isn't dead, it just smells funny* (2nd ed.). Routledge.

Sunardi, S., Yusuf, M., Gunarhadi, G., & Yeager, J. L. (2021). Inclusive education practices in Indonesian Islamic schools: Case studies of pesantren-based inclusion. *Asia Pacific Journal of Education, 41*(3), 391–405. https://doi.org/10.1080/02188791.2020.1786846

UNESCO. (2020). *Global education monitoring report: Inclusion and education—All means all*. UNESCO.

WHO. (2023). *Global report on assistive technology*. World Health Organization.

Chapter 6
Spiritual Formation and Moral Development

Abstract This chapter examines disability inclusion as a community-based process within Muslim societies, emphasizing the interconnected roles of families, mosques, and Islamic educational institutions in shaping inclusive practices. Moving beyond policy-driven approaches, the chapter argues that sustainable inclusion emerges when Islamic ethical principles are embedded within everyday social environments where values and attitudes toward disability are formed. Drawing upon Islamic moral theology, the analysis highlights concepts of human dignity (*karāmah*), justice (*ʿadl*), compassion (*raḥmah*), and collective responsibility (*farḍ kifāyah*) as normative foundations for community-driven inclusion. Empirical evidence from Indonesian contexts illustrates how cultural expectations, religious interpretations, and institutional capacities interact to either reinforce exclusion or foster participation. The chapter further explores leadership commitment, accessible infrastructure, collaborative partnerships, and stigma-reduction initiatives as mechanisms for translating theological ideals into lived social practice. By integrating contemporary inclusion theory with Islamic ethical frameworks, the chapter proposes a holistic model of community-based inclusion that positions families, religious institutions, and schools as interconnected moral actors. It concludes that sustainable disability inclusion in Muslim societies depends on aligning theological values, community engagement, and institutional accountability to create environments where all members can belong, contribute, and flourish.

Keywords Community-based Inclusion · Islamic Moral Theology · Disability Inclusion · Mosque-School Accessibility · Collective Responsibility

6.1 Introduction

Across Muslim societies, disability inclusion has increasingly become a subject of ethical, educational, and social concern. While international frameworks and national legislation have advanced disability rights and inclusive education policies,

K. Bashori, Z. Nuryana, *Disability Inclusion*, SpringerBriefs in Modern Perspectives on Disability Research,
https://doi.org/10.1007/978-981-95-8907-4_6

evidence suggests that legal reforms alone are insufficient to transform everyday experiences of persons with disabilities. Contemporary inclusion scholarship emphasizes that sustainable change depends on community participation, where social attitudes, cultural expectations, and moral commitments are shaped and reproduced (Ainscow, 2020; Slee, 2023a, 2023b). In Muslim contexts, community spaces such as families, mosques, and Islamic educational institutions carry particular significance, as they function not only as social environments but also as sites of religious learning and moral formation. Understanding disability inclusion as a community-based process is therefore essential for examining how Islamic ethical values become translated into lived practices of belonging and participation.

Islamic moral theology provides strong normative foundations for community-driven inclusion. Ethical concepts such as human dignity (*karāmah*), justice (*ʿadl*), compassion (*raḥmah*), and collective responsibility (*farḍ kifāyah*) frame social relations as interconnected moral obligations rather than individual choices (Kamali, 2021a, 2021b, 2021c, 2021d; Ghaly, 2022). From this perspective, caring for vulnerable members of society is not an act of voluntary benevolence but a shared ethical duty. Nevertheless, empirical research across Muslim-majority societies demonstrates that theological commitments to compassion often coexist with persistent stigma, limited accessibility, and exclusionary practices affecting persons with disabilities (Bazna & Hatab, 2020a, 2020b). This dissonance between moral ideals and social realities underscores the need to investigate how families, religious institutions, and schools operationalize Islamic ethics in everyday interactions.

Indonesia offers a particularly instructive context for exploring community-based inclusion within Islamic settings. As the world's largest Muslim-majority nation, Indonesia has enacted progressive disability legislation and inclusive education policies while maintaining strong religious and communal traditions (Billah et al., 2025). Despite these advances, implementation remains uneven, especially in family decision-making, mosque accessibility, and Islamic educational environments (Kurniawati et al., 2022). These dynamics illustrate how cultural norms, religious interpretations, and institutional capacity intersect in shaping opportunities for participation. Examining inclusion across family, mosque, and school contexts therefore enables a grounded understanding of how global inclusion frameworks interact with local Islamic values, communal practices, and social expectations.

Accordingly, this chapter investigates how Muslim families, mosques, Islamic schools, and community networks function as key sites for advancing inclusive participation. It analyzes leadership commitment, accessible infrastructure, collaborative partnerships, and stigma-reduction initiatives as mechanisms for embedding inclusion into community life. Drawing on Islamic ethical theory and contemporary inclusion research, the chapter frames community-based inclusion as a collective moral responsibility rather than an individual accommodation (Auda, 2021). By positioning families, religious institutions, and educational settings as interconnected moral actors, the chapter proposes a holistic model of inclusion integrating faith-based ethics with participatory social practice. Ultimately, it argues that sustainable disability inclusion in Muslim societies depends on aligning theological values, community engagement, and institutional accountability to foster environments where all members can belong, contribute, and flourish.

6.2 Inclusive Islamic Education and Spiritual Growth

Inclusive Islamic education provides a critical pathway for nurturing spiritual development among learners with disabilities by ensuring equitable access to religious knowledge, worship, and ethical formation. Within Islamic pedagogy, participation in learning the Qurʾān, practicing ritual prayer, and engaging in moral reflection are central to cultivating spiritual consciousness (*taqwā*). When students with disabilities are excluded from these processes, their opportunity for spiritual growth is constrained, contradicting Islamic ethical commitments to justice and dignity. Contemporary scholarship in inclusive education emphasizes that meaningful participation, rather than mere physical presence, is the foundation of authentic inclusion (Ainscow, 2020). Aligning this with Islamic moral theology, inclusive Islamic education affirms that every learner, regardless of ability, possesses inherent spiritual agency and the capacity for closeness to God (Kamali, 2021a, 2021b, 2021c, 2021d).

Islamic theological anthropology rejects any linkage between physical imIErment and diminished spiritual worth. The Qurʾān consistently affirms that human value is rooted in creation, not bodily or cognitive capacity (Qurʾān 17:70). Contemporary Islamic ethicists argue that dignity (*karāmah*) is unconditional and universal, extending fully to persons with disabilities (Ghaly, 2022). Inclusive religious instruction therefore becomes not simply a pedagogical adaptation but a theological necessity. When Islamic schools design accessible curricula, provide assistive supports, and adapt teaching strategies, they enact this theological principle in practice. In doing so, they affirm that learners with disabilities are not objects of charity but active participants in religious meaning-making and spiritual pursuit.

Empirical studies from inclusive Islamic schools in Indonesia demonstrate that adapted religious instruction enhances students' engagement in worship and ethical learning. Learners with disabilities who receive multisensory Qurʾānic instruction, guided prayer practice, and individualized learning plans show increased confidence, emotional stability, and sense of belonging in religious settings (Sunardi et al., 2021). These outcomes reflect broader findings in educational psychology indicating that spiritual participation contributes to resilience and positive self-concept among marginalized learners (Slee, 2023a, 2023b). Thus, inclusive Islamic education supports both cognitive access to religious content and affective connection to faith practices, forming an integrated pathway for holistic spiritual development.

Framing inclusion as a pathway to spiritual growth also reshapes how Islamic institutions understand their educational mission. Rather than viewing inclusion as an external policy requirement, it becomes an expression of *ʿibādah* (worship) and collective moral responsibility (*farḍ kifāyah*). Schools that embrace inclusive religious education cultivate communities where diversity in ability is recognized as part of divine wisdom rather than deficit (Bazna & Hatab, 2020a, 2020b). This perspective reinforces that inclusive Islamic education is not only pedagogically sound but theologically grounded, ensuring that all learners can participate in the shared pursuit of moral refinement, worship, and spiritual flourishing.

6.3 Adapted Religious Instruction and Moral Development

Adapted religious instruction in Islamic Religious Education (Pendidikan Agama Islam, IE) plays a central role in nurturing moral formation among students with disabilities. Conventional models of religious teaching often presume uniform cognitive and sensory abilities, unintentionally marginalizing learners who require alternative modes of engagement. Curriculum adaptation and multisensory pedagogies reconfigure this landscape by enabling all students to access religious concepts, ethical narratives, and ritual practices according to their capacities. Contemporary inclusive education research emphasizes that moral learning is most effective when learners can actively participate in meaning-making processes rather than passively receive instruction (Ainscow, 2020). Within Islamic pedagogy, such participation affirms students' spiritual agency (*taklīf*) and responsibility, ensuring that disability does not limit access to moral knowledge or religious experience.

Multisensory and differentiated instructional strategies further support internalization of Islamic moral values. Visual storytelling, embodied practice of prayer movements, tactile learning materials, and audio Qurʾānic recitation provide concrete pathways for students with diverse learning needs to engage with ethical teachings. These approaches align with Prophetic pedagogical traditions that emphasized demonstration, repetition, and responsiveness to individual differences (Halstead, 2004). Empirical studies from inclusive Islamic schools in Indonesia indicate that adapted IE instruction increases student engagement, reduces frustration, and strengthens behavioral consistency in daily religious practice (Nurmaliyah et al., 2023). Through these strategies, moral formation becomes an experiential process where students learn virtues such as patience, gratitude, and empathy through accessible participation.

Adapted religious instruction also cultivates ethical awareness by linking ritual practice with everyday moral conduct. Students with disabilities who actively participate in prayer, Qurʾānic recitation, and ethical reflection develop a stronger sense of belonging within the religious community. Islamic ethical scholarship emphasizes that moral accountability is not contingent upon physical or cognitive perfection but upon intention and effort (Ghaly, 2022). When educational environments honor this principle, students with disabilities are recognized as full moral agents capable of spiritual growth and ethical responsibility. Such recognition challenges deficit-based assumptions and repositions disability as part of divinely intended human diversity rather than a barrier to moral development.

Finally, the moral outcomes of adapted religious instruction extend beyond individual learners to the broader school community. Inclusive IE classrooms foster peer cooperation, mutual respect, and empathy as students learn together across differences. Contemporary moral development theory affirms that shared moral learning environments reduce prejudice and strengthen prosocial behavior (Slee, 2023a, 2023b). Within Islamic contexts, this collective learning reflects the principle of *taʿāwun* (cooperation in goodness), reinforcing communal moral bonds. Adapted religious instruction therefore functions not only as an educational strategy but as a moral intervention that shapes inclusive character formation. By aligning pedagogical practice with Islamic ethical commitments, inclusive IE contributes to spiritually grounded, morally conscious, and socially cohesive learning communities.

6.4 Empathy and Compassion in Inclusive Islamic Classrooms

Inclusive Islamic classrooms serve as vital spaces for cultivating empathy and compassion among learners. When students with and without disabilities engage together in religious learning, worship practice, and ethical reflection, they encounter human difference as a lived reality rather than an abstract concept. Contemporary inclusive education research confirms that shared learning environments reduce prejudice and promote prosocial attitudes through sustained interpersonal interaction (Ainscow, 2020; Slee, 2023a, 2023b). Within Islamic pedagogy, such encounters embody the ethical principle of *raḥmah* (mercy), which calls believers to recognize vulnerability and respond with care. Inclusive classrooms therefore function not only as sites of knowledge transmission but also as moral communities where compassionate character is formed through daily interaction.

Empirical studies from inclusive Islamic schools in Indonesia indicate that students who participate in adapted Religious Education develop stronger peer sensitivity and cooperative behavior (Qotadah et al., 2022). Group prayer activities, collaborative Qurʾānic recitation, and shared moral storytelling encourage students to support classmates with diverse learning needs. These experiences normalize interdependence and challenge dominant cultural expectations of independence and competition. Islamic ethical thought reinforces this orientation through the principle of *taʿāwun* (cooperation in goodness), positioning mutual assistance as a religious virtue (Kamali, 2021a, 2021b, 2021c, 2021d). As a result, empathy is not treated as an optional emotional trait but as a moral obligation cultivated through structured educational practice.

Inclusive classrooms also reshape how students perceive disability within their religious worldview. Rather than viewing disability through narratives of pity or deficiency, students learn to recognize classmates with disabilities as full moral and spiritual participants. Ghaly (2022) emphasizes that Islamic ethics frames human worth as independent of physical or cognitive ability, grounding interpersonal relations in dignity (*karāmah*) rather than functional capacity. When this theological principle is enacted in classroom life, students internalize respect for difference as a religious duty. Such environments reduce stigmatizing attitudes and foster compassionate peer relationships that extend beyond school into family and community interactions.

Finally, the cultivation of empathy in inclusive Islamic classrooms contributes to broader communal moral consciousness. Contemporary moral development theory highlights that ethical dispositions are strengthened when values are practiced collectively rather than taught abstractly (Slee, 2023a, 2023b). Inclusive religious learning enables students to experience solidarity, patience, and shared responsibility as part of their faith identity. In this way, inclusive education nurtures not only individual moral growth but also community transformation. By embedding compassion within pedagogical practice, Islamic schools model the Qur'ānic vision of believers as a community bound together through mercy and mutual care, reinforcing inclusion as both educational practice and spiritual commitment.

6.4.1 Spiritual Dignity, Resilience, and Self-Worth

Inclusive Islamic education nurtures psychological resilience and self-worth among learners with disabilities by grounding their identity in the Qur'ānic affirmation of inherent human dignity (*karāmah al-insān*). Islamic moral theology establishes that dignity is divinely bestowed and unconditional, independent of physical ability, cognitive capacity, or social productivity (Ghaly, 2022; Kamali, 2021a, 2021b, 2021c, 2021d). When this theological principle is embodied in classroom practice, students with disabilities encounter religious learning environments that affirm their value as full moral and spiritual agents. Such affirmation counters internalized stigma and deficit-based self-perceptions that often arise from exclusionary educational experiences. Consequently, inclusion in Islamic Religious Education does not merely facilitate access to knowledge but cultivates a stable sense of self-worth rooted in spiritual identity rather than social comparison.

Recognition of spiritual dignity also strengthens learners' capacity to cope with adversity. Disability is frequently associated with social marginalization, lowered expectations, and psychological vulnerability. However, Islamic teachings frame human trials (*balā'*) as morally meaningful experiences that do not diminish divine regard for the individual (Ghaly, 2022). When students with disabilities engage with these teachings in supportive and adapted learning environments, they develop interpretive frameworks that foster patience (*ṣabr*), hope (*rajā'*), and trust in God (*tawakkul*). These spiritual virtues contribute to emotional resilience and constructive self-understanding. Inclusive pedagogy thus mediates theological meaning in ways that transform religious narratives into psychological resources for perseverance, agency, and adaptive coping in both academic and social life.

Empirical research from inclusive Islamic schools in Indonesia indicates that recognition and participation in religious learning positively influence students' confidence and social engagement. Studies report that learners with disabilities demonstrate increased willingness to interact with peers, greater participation in collective worship, and improved self-expression when they experience acceptance and accommodation in religious classrooms (Hakiman et al., 2021; Lifshitz & Glaubman, 2002). These outcomes reflect the reciprocal relationship between dignity recognition and personal resilience: When students perceive themselves as respected contributors to a faith community, they internalize positive self-concepts.

This process also reshapes peer attitudes, generating environments where diversity is normalized and mutual respect becomes a shared moral practice rather than a charitable gesture.

From an Islamic ethical perspective, fostering resilience and self-worth among learners with disabilities is not a peripheral psychological benefit but a core moral obligation. Institutions entrusted with education bear responsibility (*masʾūliyyah*) to uphold dignity and prevent harm to learners' moral and emotional well-being (Kamali, 2021a, 2021b, 2021c, 2021d). When inclusive practices enable students with disabilities to experience belonging, recognition, and spiritual participation, educational institutions fulfill both pedagogical and ethical mandates. Resilience grounded in karāmah therefore becomes evidence of successful translation of Islamic moral theology into lived educational practice. In this sense, inclusive Islamic education contributes not only to academic access but to holistic human flourishing, where spiritual dignity sustains confidence, perseverance, and meaningful participation in community life.

6.5 Faith-Based Guidance and Behavioral Transformation

Inclusive Islamic education plays a significant role in shaping behavioral development among learners with disabilities by integrating adapted instruction in Qurʾānic ethics, ritual practice, and moral storytelling. Islamic pedagogy traditionally emphasizes character formation (*tarbiyah akhlāqiyyah*) as a central objective of religious education, positioning ethical behavior as an expression of faith rather than mere rule compliance (Halstead, 2004; Kamali, 2022). When religious instruction is adapted through multisensory methods, simplified narratives, and experiential learning, students with disabilities gain meaningful access to ethical concepts such as honesty, patience, gratitude, and responsibility. These adaptations ensure that moral instruction is internalized according to individual capacities, enabling learners to translate religious knowledge into consistent behavioral practice rather than abstract understanding alone.

Faith-based guidance further supports the development of self-regulation and emotional control. Islamic teachings on prayer (*ṣalāh*), remembrance (*dhikr*), and disciplined daily routines provide structured practices that reinforce attentional focus, impulse management, and emotional stability (Ghaly, 2022). For students with disabilities, participation in adapted ritual practices creates predictable patterns that foster psychological security and behavioral consistency. Inclusive classrooms that integrate guided prayer movements, visual sequencing of worship steps, and repetitive moral cues report improvements in students' ability to follow instructions, manage frustration, and cooperate with peers (Moordiningsih et al., 2024). Religious practice thus becomes not only spiritual engagement but also a practical mechanism for nurturing behavioral resilience and self-discipline.

Moral storytelling occupies a particularly powerful role in faith-based behavioral transformation. Qurʾānic narratives and Prophetic stories provide concrete moral exemplars that model ethical responses to adversity, injustice, and personal struggle. When these stories are presented through adapted formats, such as visual storytelling, dramatization, or tactile media, students with disabilities can engage emotionally and cognitively with moral lessons (Saksiriphol & Kunchune, 2023; Techaraungrong, 2019). Such engagement supports perspective-taking, empathy development, and reflection on personal conduct. Teachers in inclusive Islamic schools report that students exposed to adapted moral narratives demonstrate increased kindness toward peers, reduced disruptive behavior, and stronger awareness of social responsibility within classroom and community contexts.

From an Islamic ethical perspective, behavioral transformation through faith-based guidance reflects the broader aim of cultivating moral accountability (*mas'ūliyyah*) and virtuous character (*akhlāq karīmah*). Educational institutions that provide inclusive religious instruction fulfill their ethical duty to guide all learners toward responsible participation in social and spiritual life (Kamali, 2021a, 2021b, 2021c, 2021d). When students with disabilities experience consistent moral guidance in accessible formats, they develop confidence in their capacity to act ethically and contribute positively to their communities. Behavioral change, therefore, is not framed as correction of deficit but as empowerment toward moral agency. Inclusive Islamic education thus functions as a transformative space where faith-based guidance nurtures self-regulation, responsibility, and ethical maturity for every learner.

6.6 Disability as Spiritual Trial in Prophetic Tradition

Prophetic traditions (*ḥadīth*) provide a distinctive Islamic framework for understanding disability as part of divine testing (balā') and spiritual refinement rather than misfortune or deficiency. Numerous narrations describe physical imlErment, illness, or hardship as occasions through which believers attain forgiveness of sins and elevation of spiritual rank (Ghaly, 2022). These teachings construct suffering not as divine punishment but as an opportunity for moral and spiritual growth. Within Islamic pedagogy, this perspective encourages constructive meaning-making, enabling learners with disabilities to interpret personal challenges through narratives of dignity, patience, and hope. When integrated into religious education, Prophetic teachings on trial and reward cultivate positive spiritual identity rather than internalized stigma.

Central to this framework are the virtues of patience (*ṣabr*), gratitude (*shukr*), and trust in God (*tawakkul*). Prophetic guidance emphasizes that enduring hardship with patience strengthens faith and moral character (Kamali, 2021a, 2021b, 2021c, 2021d). For students with disabilities, exposure to these teachings through adapted religious instruction offers psychological reassurance and spiritual resilience. Inclusive classrooms that incorporate accessible ḥadīth narratives, reflective discussion, and guided devotional practices help learners develop coping strategies rooted in faith. Empirical studies in Islamic inclusive schools report that students who engage with such teachings display greater emotional stability, perseverance, and confidence in confronting personal limitations (Bhurawala, 2025; Qotadah et al., 2022).

Importantly, Prophetic traditions also emphasize the social responsibility of the community toward persons experiencing hardship. Narrations highlighting care for the vulnerable, hospitality toward those in need, and collective solidarity frame disability inclusion as a communal ethical duty rather than an individual burden (Bazna & Hatab, 2020a, 2020b). Teaching these traditions within inclusive religious education fosters empathy among peers and encourages shared moral responsibility. When students learn that serving and respecting persons with disabilities is an act beloved by God, inclusive attitudes become spiritually motivated rather than externally imposed. This moral framing strengthens sustainable inclusion by embedding it within religious conscience and communal identity.

From an Islamic ethical perspective, understanding disability as a spiritual trial does not justify passivity or neglect but calls for active compassion and justice. Contemporary Islamic scholars caution that the theology of trial must be coupled with ethical obligation to remove barriers and prevent harm (Ghaly, 2022). Inclusive education that draws upon Prophetic teachings therefore balances acceptance of divine wisdom with commitment to social transformation. Students with disabilities are affirmed as spiritually valued participants in the religious community, while institutions are reminded of their duty to ensure dignity and participation. Prophetic tradition thus becomes a powerful source for spiritual meaning-making, resilience, and inclusive moral consciousness.

6.7 Inclusive Spiritual Communities and Moral Flourishing

Inclusive Islamic schools and religious institutions function not only as educational spaces but also as spiritual communities where moral character and religious identity are cultivated. When such institutions intentionally embody Islamic values of dignity (*karāmah*), justice (*ʿadl*), and compassion (*raḥmah*), they create environments in which all learners, regardless of ability, experience belonging and recognition. Contemporary research in inclusive education emphasizes that participation in communal learning and worship strengthens self-worth and moral engagement among marginalized learners (Slee, 2023a, 2023b). In Islamic contexts, communal religious practice further reinforces this effect by connecting learners to shared rituals, ethical narratives, and collective responsibility. Inclusive spiritual communities thus become foundational spaces where educational participation and spiritual formation converge.

Within these environments, students with disabilities are not positioned as peripheral participants but as full members of the moral community. Islamic ethical thought affirms that communal life (*al-ḥayāh al-jamāʿiyyah*) is essential for moral development, as virtues such as empathy, patience, and cooperation emerge through relational experience (Kamali, 2021a, 2021b, 2021c, 2021d). Inclusive mosque programs, shared prayer activities, collaborative Qurʾānic study, and peer-supported religious learning provide concrete contexts for cultivating these virtues. Empirical studies from Islamic inclusive schools in Indonesia show that students who learn in such communal settings demonstrate stronger peer relationships, reduced social anxiety, and heightened moral sensitivity (Qotadah et al., 2022; Saepudin et al., 2023).

Inclusive spiritual communities also serve as powerful counterforces to stigma. When religious institutions visibly accommodate diverse bodies and learning needs, they model theological commitments to equality before God. This public embodiment of inclusion challenges deficit-based assumptions and normalizes disability as part of communal diversity rather than deviation (Bazna & Hatab, 2020a, 2020b). Regular interaction between students with and without disabilities in shared religious spaces fosters mutual recognition (*taʿāruf*) and dismantles social hierarchies based on perceived ability. Over time, these practices reshape community norms, transforming inclusion from an abstract principle into a lived moral reality.

From an Islamic moral perspective, communities that sustain inclusive participation fulfill collective responsibility (*farḍ kifāyah*) by ensuring that no member is excluded from spiritual or educational life. Such communities cultivate moral flourishing (*falāḥ*) by enabling every learner to contribute, worship, and grow according to their capacity (Ghaly, 2022). Inclusive spiritual environments therefore represent more than supportive settings; they constitute ethical ecosystems where faith, learning, and social justice intersect. By integrating Islamic moral theology with inclusive institutional practice, these communities nurture generations who embody compassion, equity, and shared spiritual excellence.

6.8 Conclusion

This chapter has demonstrated that disability inclusion in Muslim societies is most effectively realized when grounded in community-based environments shaped by Islamic moral theology and participatory social practice. Rather than relying solely on legal mandates or institutional policy reforms, sustainable inclusion emerges through everyday interactions within families, mosques, and Islamic educational institutions. Islamic ethical principles: human dignity (*karāmah*), justice (*ʿadl*), compassion (*raḥmah*), and collective responsibility (*farḍ kifāyah*) provide a normative framework that frames inclusion as a shared moral duty rather than an optional accommodation. However, empirical evidence from Muslim-majority contexts shows persistent gaps between theological ideals and lived realities, where stigma and exclusion remain embedded in cultural norms and institutional routines. Addressing these gaps requires situating inclusion within community life as a continuous ethical and social process. By examining families, religious institutions, and schools as interconnected moral actors, this chapter has highlighted how leadership commitment, accessible infrastructure, collaborative partnerships, and stigma-reduction initiatives function as practical mechanisms for embedding inclusion into communal structures. Contemporary inclusion theory affirms that community participation is essential for transforming social norms and dismantling structural barriers. When aligned with Islamic ethical commitments, these participatory processes foster environments of belonging, accessibility, and shared responsibility. Consequently, community-based inclusion becomes not only a pedagogical or social strategy but an enactment of Islamic moral accountability. Sustainable disability inclusion in Muslim societies therefore depends on integrating theological values, community engagement, and institutional stewardship to create spaces where all members are recognized, valued, and enabled to flourish.

References

Ainscow, M. (2020). Promoting inclusion and equity in education: Lessons from international experiences. *Nordic Journal of Studies in Educational Policy, 6*(1), 7–16. https://doi.org/10.1080/20020317.2020.1729583

Auda, J. (2021). *Maqāṣid al-Sharīʿah as philosophy of Islamic law: A systems approach* (2nd ed.). International Institute of Islamic Thought.

Bazna, M. S., & Hatab, T. A. (2020a). Disability in Islam: A moral framework for inclusive education. *Journal of Religion, Disability & Health, 24*(3), 287–302. https://doi.org/10.1080/15228967.2020.1751042

Bazna, M. S., & Hatab, T. A. (2020b). Disability in the Muslim world: A review of current literature. *Journal of Religion, Disability & Health, 24*(1), 1–18. https://doi.org/10.1080/15228967.2019.1701429

Bhurawala, H. (2025). Developmental and learning problems in schoolchildren: Understanding impacts on well-being in the context of Islamic schooling. In *Wellbeing in Islamic schools: Nurturing the mind, body and soul* (pp. 235–251). Springer Nature Switzerland.

Billah, M., Gassing, A. Q., Bakry, M., Kurniati, K., Haddade, A. W., Syamsuddin, D., Ahmad, L. O. I., & Harakan, A. (2025). Islamic law perspectives and social experiences on stigma toward disabled people in Indonesia. *Frontiers in Sociology, 10*, 1479243. https://doi.org/10.3389/fsoc.2025.1479243

Ghaly, M. (2022). Islamic ethics and disability: Human dignity and moral accountability. *Journal of Islamic Ethics, 6*(1), 5–24. https://doi.org/10.1163/24685542-12340060

Hakiman, H., Sumardjoko, B., & Waston, W. (2021). Religious instruction for students with autism in an inclusive primary school. *International Journal of Learning Teaching and Educational Research, 20*(12), 139–158. https://doi.org/10.26803/ijlter.20.12.9

Halstead, J. M. (2004). An Islamic concept of education. *Comparative Education, 40*(4), 517–529. https://doi.org/10.1080/0305006042000284510

Kamali, M. H. (2021a). *Equality and justice in Islam*. Islamic Texts Society.

Kamali, M. H. (2021b). *Human dignity in Islam: A foundational Islamic value*. Islamic Research Institute.

Kamali, M. H. (2021c). *Human dignity in Islam: A legal and moral framework*. Oxford University Press.

Kamali, M. H. (2021d). *Human dignity in Islam: Concept, scope, and implications*. Islamic Texts Society.

Kamali, M. H. (2022). *Maqā.ic Texts Societym: Concept, scope*. Islamic Texts Society.

Kurniawati, F., Minnaert, A., Mangunsong, F., & Ahmed, W. (2022). Inclusion in Indonesian Islamic schools: Teachers' and parents' perspectives. *International Journal of Inclusive Education, 26*(14), 1491–1507. https://doi.org/10.1080/13603116.2020.1821444

Lifshitz, H., & Glaubman, R. (2002). Religious and secular students' sense of self-efficacy and attitudes towards inclusion of pupils with intellectual disability and other types of needs. *Journal of Intellectual Disability Research, 46*(5), 405–418. https://doi.org/10.1046/j.1365-2788.2002.00424.x

Moordiningsih, M., Kristiati, A., Supartini, N., Krisnadewara, P. B., Astari, P., Agusno, M., & Mahar, H. B. P. (2024). Spiritual and community-based mental health services for children with special needs in Islamic Boarding School. *Jurnal Psikologi, 51*(1), 103–119. https://doi.org/10.22146/jpsi.89346

Nurmaliyah, Y., Aripin, S., & Nurdiansyah, N. M. (2023). 2013 curriculum: Implementation of Islamic religious education learning in schools for children with special needs. *International Journal of Islamic Thought and Humanities, 2*(1), 124–138. https://doi.org/10.54298/ijith.v2i1.83

Qotadah, H. A., Achmad, A. D., Syafri, I., Al-Anshary, A. A., & Syarifah, M. (2022). Developing student-inclusive characters through Al-Quran and 4298/i. *Khazanah Pendidikan Islam, 4*(3), 111–118. https://doi.org/10.15575/kp.v4i3.20111

Saepudin, A., Supriyadi, T., Surana, D., & Asikin, I. (2023). Strengthening character education: An action research in forming religious moderation in Islamic education. *International Journal of Learning Teaching and Educational Research, 22*(12), 84–105. https://doi.org/10.26803/ijlter.22.12.5

Saksiriphol, D., & Kunchune, P. (2023). Development of picture storytelling books to enhance morality and word reading ability of special needs students in Thailand. *International Journal of Instruction, 16*(3), 245–260. https://doi.org/10.29333/iji.2023.16314a

Slee, R. (2023a). *Inclusive education isn't dead, it just smells funny*. Routledge.

Slee, R. (2023b). Inclusive education isn't dead, it just smells funny. *Discourse: Studies in the Cultural Politics of Education, 44*(1), 1–15. https://doi.org/10.1080/01596306.2022.2142594

Sunardi, S., Yusuf, M., Kurniawati, F., & Marlina, M. (2021). Inclusive Islamic schools in Indonesia: Practices, challenges, and innovations. *International Journal of Inclusive Education, 25*(9), 1051–1068. https://doi.org/10.1080/13603116.2020.1748610

Techaraungrong, P. (2019). The development of storytelling multimedia book for promotion of the moral and ethics for hearing impaired students. In *Proceedings of the 2019 5th International Conference on Education and Training Technologies* (pp. 73–77). https://doi.org/10.1145/3337682.3337688

MIX
Papier aus verantwortungsvollen Quellen
Paper from responsible sources
FSC® C105338

FSC
www.fsc.org

If you have any concerns about our products,
you can contact us on
ProductSafety@springernature.com

In case Publisher is established outside the EU,
the EU authorized representative is:
Springer Nature Customer Service Center GmbH
Europaplatz 3, 69115 Heidelberg, Germany

Printed by Libri Plureos GmbH
in Hamburg, Germany